FULL REVII
BUILT TO THRIVE

Dr. Shelly Sethi is an expert Integrative Medicine physician who offers up the best basic principles of integrative medical advice in a captivating and straightforward way. Her wisdom, grounded in both personal and professional experience and offers readers the key fundamentals for the first steps into a lifelong journey into better health and wellness. While the journey is not easy in our current culture, Dr. Sethi makes the core components available to her readers in attainable manner. There are many "how-to" books out there, and this is one of my favorites for the first steps into better health.

ANN MARIE CHIASSON, MD
INTERIM DIRECTOR, FELLOWSHIP IN INTEGRATIVE MEDICINE
ARIZONA CENTER FOR INTEGRATIVE MEDICINE
UNIVERSITY OF ARIZONA, TUCSON, ARIZONA
AUTHOR OF *ENERGY HEALING: THE ESSENTIALS OF SELF-CARE*

A rising star in the field of integrative health and medicine, Dr. Shelly Sethi provides a beautiful and inspiring vision of how we can manifest a life that nourishes and strengthens our bodies, minds and spirits. The title says it all: Built to Thrive is a blueprint for wellbeing in the 21st century. I highly recommend it.

TIERAONA LOW DOG, MD
AUTHOR: *NATIONAL GEOGRAPHIC'S LIFE IS YOUR BEST MEDICINE*

Built to Thrive is a simple, strategic, and soulful journey to self-discovery. Dr. Sethi has incorporated time-tested strategies that are evidenced and supported by modern research to help readers live their best life, a life where families and communities thrive. Dr. Sethi places a great deal of emphasis on the power of food, environment, and self-love. This book is your guide to living the way your creator intended. It's your time to thrive!

SACHIN PATEL, DC
FOUNDER OF THE LIVING PROOF INSTITUTE
AUTHOR OF *PERFECT PRACTICE*

BUILT
TO
THRIVE

DR SHELLY SETHI

BUILT
TO
THRIVE

Overcome Chronic Illness, Fatigue and Hormonal
Imbalance and Get Your Energy and Vitality Back
Without Medication or Surgery

9 DOCTOR PROVEN STRATEGIES

DR SHELLY SETHI

Disclaimer

This book is designed as a reference and is made available to the public with the understanding that the author and the publisher are not rendering medical or other professional advice tailored to individual needs and situations. You should not use the information contained in this book as a substitute for the advice of a licensed health-care professional and should consult a health-care professional to address any health concerns specific to you.

Because nutritional supplements can interact with medications or affect some medical conditions, you should always check with your prescribing health-care professional before using the herbal remedies described in this book.

The author and publisher disclaim any liability whatsoever with respect to any loss, injury, or damage arising out of the use of the information contained in this book or omission from any information in this book. Mention of specific products, companies, or organizations does not imply that the publisher and author of this book endorse such products, companies, or organizations.

Additional books may be ordered through http//www.drshellysethi.com or by contacting us at drsethi@drshellysethi.com

Because of the dynamic nature of the Internet, web addresses or links contained in this book may have changed since publication and may no longer be valid.

DEDICATION AND GRATITUDE

I gratefully dedicate this book to my beloved little boys, Viren and Dhruv, who inspire me every day to live in the present moment. They remind me to laugh at both the small things and the big. Additionally, without the support and encouragement of my husband, Bobby, this book would not have been possible. He is also the one who taught me how to take life less seriously. I am forever grateful for unwavering love from my parents. Although he doesn't know it, my father, Raj Sethi, is the reason for my journey into medicine and wellness and the one who keeps me inspired to keep discovering. It is my mother, Dipy Sethi, however that has shown me the power of the heart and how to know spirit within. She is also the creator of the most delicious and nourishing food that I have ever eaten. My love of healing spices, fresh vegetables and cooking comes from my mother and my grandmothers, Kaushalya Devi Sethi and Satyavati Kapoor. I still dream of peeling peas with my grandmother at her kitchen table. I am additionally grateful to my sisters, Pooja Sethi and Sonali Sethi, my brother-in-law, Vivek Kulkarni and my in-laws, Pat and Bob Harding for all the help and support these last few years that allowed me the opportunity to travel and learn and write.

I would also like to thank my mentors and teachers along the way. Specifically, Dr. Andrew Weil, Dr. Victoria Maizes,

Dr. Hilary McClafferty and others at the Arizona Center for Integrative Medicine. Dr. Ann Marie Chiasson helped me rediscover ceremony and remember to trust my intuition through energy medicine which has been an invaluable part of my growth. Dr. Tieraona Low Dog has shown me the beauty of plant medicine and I am forever grateful.

Lastly and most importantly, I thank my spiritual guides and teachers who have helped me see my truth.

Table of Contents

INTRODUCTION:
THE WHY

You're looking in the mirror. What do you see? Do you see a happy, healthy person who's fulfilling her dreams? Or someone you don't recognize and aren't sure you want to be? Imagine passing by that mirror and recognizing the person looking back at you. Imagine seeing a woman who has energy to do everything she wants that day. Imagine knowing that the choices you make every single day make a difference in how you look and feel. Imagine maintaining your energy as you age, sustaining your ability to think clearly and make a difference, and being the best you at every stage of your life.

This is what I'd love to see you discover. And I know it's possible for you, just as it was possible for the hundreds of patients I've worked with in my clinic. Having worked with these people, I've seen a pattern and discovered a process that works to heal them and keep them well.

It's the reason I wrote this book. It's the reason I'm right here right now. You'll meet one of these patients in a moment, but first let me go back to where it all started and why I chose this path.

For as long as I can remember, I asked a lot of whys. In fact, I asked "why?" so often that my aunt finally bought me the *Big Book of Why* in hopes that I would find my answers there and give her some peace. When I was very young, I used to spend my summers in India, a country filled with mysticism, in-your-face poverty and the richness of spirit. I would beg my aunt and my parents to take me to the temple where the old yoga masters were teaching meditation and yoga. I listened earnestly to their teachings hoping that they could answer some of my whys. I would ask my uncle to take me to the little bookstore in the crowded marketplace in central Delhi by his office. There, I would meet the old bookseller, and he would take out his ladder, climb up the dusty bookshelves, and pull down a stack of spiritual books for me to read. Apparently, I was the youngest person ever to buy those books from him, not that I had much competition for them. I devoured the books with the same intensity that I devoured mango ice cream on those chokingly hot summer days without air conditioning. I was convinced that the sacred texts describing the union of the mind and the body, the spirit and emotion, and food and health would give me clues that would help me answer the questions that continued to nag away at me: "Why am I here?" and "What is my purpose?"

During those summers in India, I was exposed to many different traditions and rich cultural inheritances through my grandmother. She often used spices and herbs to fix ailments. For example, we were fed concoctions of turmeric, ginger, honey, and lemon juice for a cough. A tummy ache was treated with ingested peppermint oil, and a tea made from fennel seeds and ajwain seeds. Rarely did the doctor show up at our home. If and when he did, his treatment consisted of some sort of injection along with a number of homeopathic or Ayurvedic remedies. If you're unfamiliar with Ayurvedic Medicine, let me explain briefly. Ayurveda is one of the first systems of medicine originating over 3000 years ago. It is based on the belief that the balance between body, mind and spirit is the root of health and wellness. It is a practice that takes into account an individual's makeup, and recommends lifestyle modifications that promote good health not just treat disease.

Cuts and bruises were often treated by my grandmother as well. She would take half an onion, cut crisscrosses into it, sprinkle it with a bright golden spice and tie it to the wound. I don't know if this sped up healing or not, but I can attest to my skin turning yellow. As a physician, I have read many published studies, over the years, about that golden spice: turmeric. I've learned how it actually does help with inflammation. It has a number of antimicrobial properties as well, and stimulates the immune system to heal.

As I grew older, I became more interested in the mind-body practices of healing. My father was the catalyst that set me on that career path, but I'm ahead of myself. First came high school and my freshman year, which was when I discovered meditation and started practicing it daily for hours on end. Because I was introduced to spiritual healers and exposed to such teachings during my youth in India, I took up meditation with gusto. I'd wake up at 4:00 in the morning and sit in meditation until 6:00 or 7:00. My meditation often ended with my mother banging on my door asking what I was doing in my room. She had a running fear that I would somehow decide I was too spiritual for this world, and would run off to the Himalayas and become an ascetic. An ascetic is a person who gives up the worldly life in pursuit of spiritual growth.

When I entered college, I had no intention of being a physician. I was however, fascinated by the healing arts and quantum physics. I read Deepak Chopra's *Quantum Healing* and Dr. Andrew Weil's *Optimal Eating for Optimal Health*. I already knew about the importance of good nutrition for health, but this was the first time I was introduced to the scientific methods around stress affecting physiology and health.

In the midst of learning and absorbing these concepts, I got a call from my sister during the summer prior to entering my junior year of college. I was studying with a professor who was investigating chronic illness and the effects of stress on the body. My sister informed me that my dad, unknown to me, was experiencing typical angina-like symptoms and had been for many months. He had become very ill, after it was misdiagnosed initially as acid reflux. Luckily for him, my older sister was in medical school. When he told her about his symptoms, she immediately called in a favor and got one of the attending cardiologists to evaluate him. Essentially, the cardiologist told him he must stay in hospital and wasn't allowed home. His heart was in such bad condition that they needed to operate the day after he was admitted. He had a number of blockages in his heart vessels and needed open-heart surgery.

My world turned upside down. I didn't understand how a seemingly healthy person could suddenly be minutes away from maybe dying. In hindsight, this should not have been a surprise. My father was obese, and had been diagnosed with diabetes a few years earlier. Like many typical south Asian males, his diet contained way too many simple carbohydrates. He had immigrated to the USA in the early 1970s alone to advance his chemical engineering career. He was a type A, high-stress person and didn't manage that stress well, nor did he have any tools to combat the daily pressures of life in America. This was also a time when signals from doctors, corporations and the health industry gave out conflicting information about nutrition.

I had watched my father go on yo-yo diets to lose weight. There were weeks when I'd come home to the sulfurous smell of stewing cabbages because he was on The Cabbage Soup Diet. His typical breakfast was cereal. He followed what, at the time, was thought to be good medical advice. He maintained a low-fat yet high-carbohydrate diet. Now we know better!

Six bypasses later, my father made it through those surgical procedures and was again told to maintain a low-fat diet because "it would be best for his health". He went on to have progression of heart disease, macular degeneration, diabetic neuropathy, and bilateral knee replacements (due to the weight). Naturally, he never got the weight down in a sustainable way.

I began to question if there was some way to prevent his type of suffering. How does someone get themselves into a position where another human being has to crack open their chest? Why would anyone put their heart at the mercy of a surgeon's hands? There had to be some way to stop this from happening. *This can't possibly be the unavoidable fate of humans as they age*, I thought. I couldn't help reflecting on the emotional and energetic consequences of this experience and how disempowered my father must have felt. Did the master life-giving organ fail spontaneously or did he miss its warning cries for help? Was he destined to succumb to his genes or did his life choices contribute to the process of disease creation? Unfortunately for my father, he lost his own dad when he was only three years old. His mother was so traumatized by the loss she experienced that she was unable to share any health history about his father with him. In fact, my grandmother realized early on that the only way for my father to escape the trauma and the poverty that she was forced to succumb to after the loss of her husband was through an education. This guiding principle shaped the rest of his life and every choice he made was driven by the desire to have financial freedom, and unlimited access to food. Food became the emotional Band-Aid, the celebratory prize to a lifetime dedicated to overcoming poverty and finally having it all. There was never a shortage of food on the dinner table and it was mandatory to finish what we were given on our plate followed by a large glass of milk because "there were children starving in India". Fragrant white basmati rice or puffed wheat roti (similar to a tortilla) were served with every Indian-style meal and bread with every American-style meal. This was a sign of prosperity that my family clung to. We often had meatloaf or pasta with beef bolognese, even though neither beef nor pasta is typically consumed in India. The ability to eat red meat and experience the cuisines of the world were some of the ways in which my parents adapted to their new American lifestyle. When we traveled, McDonald's fried fish sandwiches, or Big Mac with fries followed by apple pie in a box were our staples. Unbeknownst to us, these inflammatory foods, coupled with a work ethic that created chronic underlying stress and little time for exercise or rest, was slowly clogging my dad's arteries, expanding his belly, and causing his hormones and insulin to become unbalanced. Over a couple of decades, without any meaningful advice otherwise from his doctors, this lifestyle of indulging in food and work to overcome that which his childhood lacked resulted in my father lying on an operating table before the age of 50 with his ribs spread apart, and a stranger's gloved hands embracing his lifegiving organ.

The experience of our family during my father's unwellness was the catalyst for me realizing what I wanted to do with my life. Somehow, I had to figure why this happened to him and what I could do about it. As I read and researched, my desire to educate about prevention grew. I realized that prevention also meant healing from the subconscious and unconscious messages that are formed in childhood that play in our mind over and over, sabotaging our ability to make real and sustainable change. The medicine I experienced as a child during my frequent trips to India was not centered on drugs and pills or surgery. It included the use of healing spices, botanicals and plants, yoga for movement and cleansing the body, and ultimately caring for the mind and spirit through meditation. This was my definition of a healer. On that summer afternoon of my freshman year of college, with my ear on the receiving end listening to the terrible news my sister was sharing, I saw my future with crystal clarity.

I chose to attend medical school as I truly believed I would learn to be a healer there. In hindsight, instead of becoming the holistic healer I strove to become, medical school shaped me into a disease-focused physician with limited tools to help my patients. This came as great news to my father, because as any typical southeast Asian child knows, there are only three professions that parents of my father's generation find desirable: doctor, lawyer, or engineer.

While in osteopathic medical school, I learned how to use my hands to feel the fascia and connectedness of the body. I discovered that sometimes the body presents a symptom (such as back pain or muscle tightness) that is actually a reflection of what's going on internally. Back pain, for example, may not just be back pain. It might be the body screaming that the gut is unhealthy, or that the gallbladder is obstructed. Pain in the body can also reflect unaddressed emotions that manifest as chronic underlying stress, which causes inflammation and results in pain.

Throughout my training, I sought out and studied with as many "alternative" medical practitioners as I could. I studied traditional Chinese medicine, Ayurvedic medicine, herbal medicine, and aromatherapy in addition to all kinds of interesting healing modalities including energy medicine.

When I completed my training, I took a position in a fairly conventional family medicine practice at a clinic. I had about seven to ten minutes to spend with each patient after the nurse was done taking their vitals and entering all the data into a computer. In this allotted time, I was supposed to hear their story, connect with them on an emotional level, diagnose their condition, come up with a treatment plan, and explain it all to them. I became increasingly frustrated. I felt that my true intentions and the reasons for wanting to become a physician in the first place were getting further and further away from me.

After some time, I decided to complete fellowship training in integrative medicine through the Arizona Center for Integrative Medicine. I was fortunate to study with my initial mentor, Dr. Andrew Weil. During the fellowship, I learned about the mounting evidence on how herbal remedies cured ailments, supporting many of the non-Western modalities I was exposed to as a young child in India. For example, the turmeric that my grandmother put on an onion and applied to our wounds had been found to be a powerful anti-inflammatory treatment. I learned how certain spices, such as black pepper and turmeric, combine to increase the potency and availability of the healing properties of those foods. In India, we always combine turmeric and black pepper; it is a recipe for healing foods that has been passed down for centuries. And I learned how meditation, which I began in ninth grade, was actually transforming my brain by a process called neuroplasticity.

Various studies support how connection to community and spirituality improves our lives and health while reducing illness.

All this learning was exciting for me. I finally felt I was rediscovering the truths that I had always known. I knew we each had the power to shape our health. I have filled my toolbox with healing modalities that address not just the physical body which manifests disease, but also the emotional and spiritual bodies that are often at the root of chronic illness. These tools are accessible to anyone and everyone. They can be applied in any situation, whether you are struggling to overcome a condition you have had for years, or you just want to be sure you are optimizing and living your fullest life.

I wrote this book to get you started on your journey. I wrote this book so that you remember that you were built to thrive. As I said in the beginning, I wrote this book so that you can join the hundreds of patients who have already achieved their version of thriving after working with me in my practice.

What might that look like? Allow me to introduce you to one such patient — Katie. Five years ago, Katie did not feel the way she does now. Back then, she had low energy, couldn't concentrate because of the constant brain fog and found it difficult to shift those last few stubborn pounds. She had taken too many sick days at work, so her income had taken a tumble. Her relationship was suffering because her hormones were all over the place, and her libido was nowhere to be seen. And she felt exhausted and sad that she was often so tired she couldn't enjoy spending time with her children or friends. If she went out to dinner, she would feel bloated and uncomfortable in herself. And lately she'd noticed her skin was looking worse, seeing blemishes more of the time.

When Katie came to me, she'd had enough and was ready to commit to doing everything she could to change her health for the better. Together, we used the tools and information I'm going to share with you in this book, and she took back her life. Here's what that looked like. First, when Katie started working with us, we did in-depth lab tests. We found she had a small intestinal bowel overgrowth, an imbalance in her natural gut bacteria, and her digestive enzymes were low so she was not absorbing nutrients of food. We worked with targeted support using supplements and botanicals to decrease overgrowth and restore balance. As Katie's issues began to clear and the inflammation in her digestive system decreased, she also noticed that her acne disappeared and she could add foods back into her diet. Most importantly, her confidence grew and she felt excited about her days again, because working together on her health gave her back her energy. She was happier and more satisfied at work (not to mention being more effective and feeling less guilty), and when she got home, she still had some energy to be the kind of mom she wanted to be for her kids, the kind of wife she wanted to be to her husband and the kind of friend she wanted to be for her friends. So although the focus of our work together was the physical changes to her health, like balancing her hormones and reducing the stress on her system as a whole, what really transformed was her purpose, drive and desire to create loving relationships with the people who mattered to her.

What's special about Katie's story is there's nothing special about Katie's story. Simply, she was ready and committed to herself and to doing the work she needed to do to thrive in her life again. And that's available to everyone. It's available to you. By reading and applying all that I'm going to teach you in *Built To Thrive*, you too can see the same results.

Sadly, some people believe they can't change, that they were born with the wrong genes, that their fate is predetermined. Others believe that medication alone will fix all their troubles.

These people are not part of our practice and they won't get what they're looking for here.

Built To Thrive will allow you to review your lifestyle, including how you sleep, how you move, what you eat, how you connect, how you are living your purpose and how you deal with stress. You will get detailed information and a roadmap to restoring your body to its natural best health. You'll get specific ways to heal and recover your body on a cellular, energetic, spiritual and emotional level.

You too can feel increased energy, improved mood and motivation to live your life the way you want. You too can open up opportunities for increased satisfaction and reward for your work, and greater connection with your family and friends. It's possible. I've seen it. And you deserve it.

Take it from me… Don't leave it until emergency heart surgery is your only option. Nobody deserves that. You were made to be healthy and happy. And this is your chance to grasp your health and happiness, and hold onto it. Having seen the impact of ill-health on my family and countless families who have come to me, I understand what you are going through and am committed to helping people just like you. I have witnessed the healing that can happen in the body, mind and spirit when given the right tools.

Throughout this book, you will find many recommendations and resources. I hope you will practice using the tools included here to help you heal at the root of chronic illness, hormonal imbalance, and low energy. If you are feeling good already, these tools and principles can be directed towards building a foundation for a sustainable lifestyle that will keep you feeling vital and energetic. Prevention is the key word here.

Built To Thrive will guide you in making lifestyle choices that will help you take back your health: because your health belongs to you, and not to our healthcare system!

1

NUTRITION FOR NOURISHMENT

"Eat food, not too much,
mostly plants."

~ MICHAEL POLLAN

Wherever I go, one of the main questions I get asked is: What is the right diet for me? This is a difficult question to answer in some ways. There are *so many diets* out on the market... It seems as though every few months somebody has come up with a new diet. A brand new, never before seen, guaranteed to work diet. While this may seem appealing, many of these diets are actually the same in failing to be tailored to you and the biological factors that are unique to you as I will discuss in the next few paragraphs. Additionally, too much conflicting information can be confusing and overwhelming.

You may well wonder: *What does all this mean? What's the correct plan for me? Paleo or plant-based? Or would going vegan be the kind of diet that would decrease the manifestation of chronic disease?* Truth be told, it just depends. It depends on your genetic predisposition, the make-up of the gut bacteria that live inside you and break your food down, as well as the health of your gut, and other factors. The good news is that a general goal and principle of sound nutrition is to feed your body essential nutrients while not potentiating the inflammatory response in your body. What I mean by this is that certain foods will provide little to no nutritional value, meanwhile acting as a source of stress for the body. Usually, foods that do this are not natural or real whole foods, but rather ones that have been created or processed in a factory. Therefore, a consistent way to reduce the inflammatory response in the body is to eliminate processed foods and refined sugars.

Additionally, there are foods that quickly turn into sugar in your body. These foods are considered high on the glycemic index scale. The glycemic index is a relative ranking of carbohydrate in foods according to how they affect blood glucose levels. Carbohydrates with a low glycemic index (55 or less) are more slowly digested, absorbed and metabolized. They cause a lower and slower rise in blood glucose and, therefore, usually, insulin levels. This is not a perfect system or measure of how individual foods will react in your body; however, it is a good place to begin understanding how to evaluate the foods in your current diet. Some limitations of the glycemic index are that the index can be affected by other foods that you eat at the same time. For example, though pasta ranks high on the glycemic index scale and quickly increases your blood sugar levels after eating, if it is combined with an acid such as vinegar in a tomato sauce, this slows the release of the sugar into your bloodstream. Learning about food-combining to optimize your diet can be fun and beneficial.

"PERFECTION" VERSUS PRINCIPLES

With these principles in mind from the start, it's important to note before we continue that the purpose of this chapter is not to come up with the "perfect diet" because the perfect diet doesn't exist. Rather, I want to empower you to understand how food and nutrition affects your health and how it can be a first line of defense against developing disease or halting its progress.

Nutritional science has changed a lot over the years. We continue to isolate nutrients or food groups and look for evidence of harm or benefit. This is a reductionist view of food. The truth is we will never be able to create the perfect research study on how a particular food affects us. This is because our bodies are complex. We each have a particular set of genetic information that we are born with; then layer on top of that the makeup of the organisms within our gut that help us break down our food. The variety of gut bugs we each have is determined by many factors including where we grew up, how we came into the world, via C-section or via the birth canal, and whether or not we nursed or were bottle-fed.

Additionally, the environment in which we live and the day-to-day exposures we have to various toxins also interact with our genetics and our particular makeup of gut organisms. We are exposed to many chemicals in the air we breathe, the water we drink, the dirt on our food and even in our food. So, we eat food, and this food interacts with our body through the genes that we have, the microbes that we house and the chemicals that burden our bodies. You can imagine the difficulty even the most highly trained nutritionist would have in answering the question:

What is the right diet for you?

As I mentioned at the start of this chapter, the answer is it depends on all those factors and more.

There are, however, some nutritionally sound principles that apply to most everyone. Thank goodness for that! Based on current nutritional science, the following is most likely applicable:

In the Western world, we eat way *too many processed foods* and simple sugars. The link between eating processed foods and sugar and the occurrence of chronic diseases including diabetes, heart disease, obesity, autoimmune conditions, and cancer is increasing tremendously.

A particular diet that might be right for one person may not be the answer for another. However, a *generalized anti-inflammatory eating regimen* seems to benefit the majority of people.

The diet that has the most evidence in support of reducing long-term chronic disease is The Mediterranean Diet or the anti-inflammatory diet. Let's discuss that. Many studies conducted globally produced evidence in support of The Mediterranean Diet, where people typically eat a plant-based diet with some components of clean sources of animal protein, mostly seafood. People who eat this type of diet tend to have fewer illnesses and less chronic disease. A wellexplored example of this are the Blue Zones: areas of the world where the most centurions live. In studying these areas of the world, researchers note that these people have many things in common, one of them being eating habits. Typically, their diet consists of mostly fresh plants and vegetables. Usually there are little-to-no pesticides or chemicals in the farming process. Good sources of fish with high amounts of omega-3 fatty acids are included in their diet. Limited amounts of animal protein are found, yet if they do eat animal meat, it originates from grass-fed or pasture-raised animals.

What is not found in their diet? Large amounts of simple sugars, processed foods, chemical-laden drinks and sodas, dairy that has been injected with growth hormones and antibiotics. It appears there are no genetically modified foods (GMOs) or high amounts of GMO corn and gluten. Their diet includes a variety of fruits and vegetables, whole grains, lots of nuts and seeds, and occasionally red wine.

EAT REAL FOOD

When I discuss nutrition and dietary habits with my patients, we focus on real food. Real food is simply food that your grandmother would recognize as food: as close as you can get to how it is found in nature, not processed or created in a factory or lab.

A particular dietary plan may vary, based on the individual. This may include the elimination of a particular type of food not suited to the individual based on their genetics, metabolism or current state of health. This is where the personalized nutritional evaluation becomes handy. If you are working with an integrative or functional medicine physician, you may have a specific dietary plan that's been prescribed for you. If you haven't been given a particular dietary plan, then incorporating an anti-inflammatory diet or The Mediterranean Diet is a good place to start. It's also a long-term sustainable dietary plan for your family. You can find more information on this diet here: **https://www.drweil.com/diet-nutrition/antiinflammatory-diet-pyramid/dr-weils-anti-inflammatory-diet/**

DIETARY POINTERS

I have spent the last few years studying nutrition. As this science evolves, I've found that some recommendations remain consistent. Here is a list of general guidelines to follow when choosing your food:

1. Eat as much organic food as possible. If you are on a budget, I recommend following the Dirty Dozen and Clean Fifteen list. This list incorporates the foods that tend to have the highest amount of pesticides in them. As a rule of thumb, if a fruit or vegetable is thinskinned and brightly colored, it typically has a high amount of pesticides. This is because insects and other species are attracted to those types of fruits and vegetables, so pesticides are used as a deterrent. The Environmental Working Group has a printable resource that you can take to the grocery store as a reminder. The list can be found here: **https://www.ewg.org/foodnews/dirty_dozen_list**

2. When purchasing dairy, be sure the products are free from growth hormones, antibiotics, and if at all possible, are grass-fed or pasture-raised. This is because you will ingest all the chemicals that were given to those cows. It has been proven that the higher use of antibiotics in dairy animals has increased the resistance to antibiotics in humans. It has also greatly shifted the microbiome. The microbiome is that collection of various microbes, bacteria, and other species that live on and within you, which I referred to earlier when discussing gut health. When you ingest foods that contain antibiotics, you kill off some of the highly beneficial microbes and bacteria that are there to protect you.

This can greatly affect your health.

3. When choosing seafood, choose fish that is low in mercury and preferably wild caught. If you are unable to purchase wild caught seafood, the second-best option is sustainably farmed fish. Trout and salmon are found in this category. There is mounting evidence that fish from China and Vietnam (where much of the industry exports their fish for packaging) is laden with mercury or impure. Mercury tends to accumulate in fish that are large and fatty such as tuna, yellowtail and other varieties. Mercury and other heavy metals are neurotoxins that affect the brain as well as overall health. A neurotoxin is a poisonous substance that acts on the brain and the nervous system and disrupts communication. A general rule of thumb for choosing fish low in mercury is: the smaller the fish, the more likely it is to have a lower mercury content. Fish such as herring, sardines, river salmon, and black cod are excellent choices to include in your diet. Not only are they low in mercury, but they also have high amounts of omega-3 fatty acids. Omega-3 fatty acids are potent anti-inflammatory molecules that are beneficial to humans in many ways. These fatty acids support brain growth and development.

Although it's important to try to find fish that is wild caught, take note that humans are overfishing many species. Some of them may cease to exist in our waters in the near future. A good source to check is the list of sustainable fish at http://www.seafoodwatch.org. This organization also has an app that can be loaded onto your phone for quick reference at the grocery store or fish market.

4. Reduce the amount of processed flour in your diet. Any time a grain is processed into a flour, it is more likely to turn quickly into sugar in the body. By reducing the amount of foods in your diet that turn quickly into sugar, you'll automatically reduce the up and down blood sugar response which causes insulin to spike and drop. Refined flour is a major cause of inflammation in the body and can lead to diabetes down the road, as well as hormonal imbalance. Sadly, the list of foods that contain refined flour includes pancakes, muffins, cakes, cookies, and for that matter, any type of bread. I have found a variety of products available on the market made from ground nut flours. These can be an alternative choice and many recipes feature nut flours for baking.

5. Choose water or teas as your beverage of choice. We have an unhealthy love affair with soda, and juices are all too often included in our diet. These beverages become a quick source of sugar for the body and cause insulin spikes and rapid drops in blood sugar. This affects your overall energy and balance, and can cause fatigue and afternoon crashes.

6. Try intermittent fasting. Giving your body some time to rest from digestion is quite beneficial. From an evolutionary standpoint, the human species has had times of feast and famine. In modern times, people are frequently eating between large meals and overeating at mealtimes. In order to understand how intermittent fasting can benefit you, you need to understand the difference between two states of being: the fed state and the fasted state. Let's pretend you begin eating a

meal. From the time you begin eating until about three to five hours later, your body is focused on digestion and absorption. During this time, your insulin levels rise in order to deal with the incoming sugar from the food you just ate. When insulin levels are high, the body typically doesn't need to burn fat for energy, because you have a supply of energy coming in from your food. Following the three to five hour time period, your body enters a period of time where is it not digesting, but is also not fasted. This is called the post-absorptive state. You then enter the fasted state and insulin levels drop. Now your body begins to burn fat for energy. Now suppose you eat snacks or drink soda or juice before you enter the fasted states. Well, then the insulin levels go right back up and you never entered the fat-burning state. Fasting allows your body to enter a fat-burning state typically not achieved with a normal eating schedule. Recent evidence shows that abstention from eating for somewhere between 13 and 16 hours, allows your body to reset and get back to a fasted or rested phase. Intermittent fasting may be a factor in cancer prevention as well. I suggest ending dinner around 7:00 PM and then eating again the following morning at 8:00 or 9:00 AM. You can, of course, adjust this start and end time as you need to, based on your lifestyle.

7. Include cruciferous vegetables in your diet daily unless you cannot tolerate green, crunchy and leafy vegetables, such as broccoli, cauliflower, or kale. This group of vegetables contains a compound called sulforaphane. Sulforaphane helps prevent cancer by acting as a detoxifier of chemicals that are taken into

the body. Eating cruciferae on a daily basis can reduce the risk of developing breast or prostate cancer. It has other beneficial metabolic effects in the body and helps hormonal balance by decreasing blood sugar and decreasing obesity. So basically, cruciferae are a powerhouse set of vegetables that fight cancer, help prevent diabetes and make you less fat. There's a quick recipe for roasted cauliflower with herbs in the final chapter of the book. You can find more recipes like this on my website here: https://www.drshellysethi.com/recipes

8. Include nuts, seeds and other good fats in your diet liberally. Nuts and seeds are a wonderful source of omega-3 fatty acids, as are olive oil and avocados. Olive oil is best eaten raw by drizzling it on your food or adding it to a cooked dish once it's out of the oven or pan.

9. Eat a colorful variety of fruits and vegetables every single day. Eating a rainbow of vegetables gives diversity to our microbiome. The greater the diversity of your microbiome and the microbes that live within you, the healthier you'll be. Depending on their color, vegetables or fruit have different beneficial nutrients such as antioxidants or vitamins. Eating a proper serving of them is important to help prevent cancer, autoimmune disease, and other chronic illnesses. This will ensure that you are obtaining the variety of health-benefiting nutrients that you need.

10. Eat real food.

GUT HEALTH: WORST OFFENDERS AND BEST BETS

These are four of the worst offenders for decreasing gut microbiome diversity:

1. Medication usage, the most harmful being antibiotics and proton-pump inhibitors (used to treat heartburn).

2. A high-calorie diet, high in simple carbohydrates (such as candy, white breads, white pasta, baked sweets etc).

3. Frequent eating - turns out eating small meals every two hours (grazing) is not ideal for our gut microbiome.

4. Sweetened drinks, such as soda and juices with added sugar and high fructose corn syrup.

And here are the five top ways to improve gut microbiome diversity:

1. Ensuring a high-fiber diet of whole vegetables and fruits.

2. Eating dark chocolate

3. Including fermented foods in your diet, like yogurt, miso, sauerkraut, kimchi.

4. Consuming some red wine.

5. Drinking plenty of green tea.

In addition to those foods found in the research studies, here are a couple of actions you can take to improve the variety of good bugs in your gut.

1. **Take a good quality probiotic.** It should be a reputable brand and have a good variety of both lactobacillus and *bifidobacterium*. Until we have more specific data on which exact strains are helpful, this is a good rule of thumb.

2. **Provide prebiotic food for the bacteria.** Prebiotics are the non-digestible food that the bacteria need to thrive. These include fiber, oligofructose and inulin found in the skin of apples, bananas, onions, garlic, Jerusalem artichoke, chicory root and beans. You can also get a prebiotic supplement or try potato starch in a smoothie.

2

SLEEP AND REST

"To achieve the impossible dream,
try going to sleep."

~ JOAN KLEMPNER

In medical school, we spent little time getting sleep, let alone learning about it. Though it was cursorily alluded to that it was an important part of well-being, there was no discussion around what actually happens within and to the body during sleep. Since that time, and due to advancements in technology, including the ability to monitor the brain during sleep, we've been able to understand the many crucial processes that occur during sleep, without which we would die.

Sleep is a time when we integrate everything that has happened in our waking lives: from our environmental experiences: conscious, subconscious and unconscious, to all the visual and auditory inputs, plus the often-overlooked olfactory input. Everything that you think, hear, smell, see, and taste becomes integrated into your understanding of the world. It all gets processed during sleep. Sleep offers us the chance to wake up with a new understanding and perception of how we operate.

Dreams and the recall of dreams can have a profound effect on how we process our emotions. When we remember our dreams, it can provide insight into the unresolved situations in our life that cause us worry, depression, anger or rage. These feelings often go unacknowledged and ignored. Dreams may have trivial or significant meaning attached to them.

SLEEP CYCLES

A variety of processes happen throughout the different stages of sleep. We typically go through four cycles of sleep, plus an REM cycle. Each of these stages has a different purpose.

Stage 1 is a light cycle of sleep. Here our brain is producing alpha and beta waves, and our eye movements slow down. Typically, this stage is fairly brief, lasting around seven minutes or so. In stage 1, we are somewhat alert and can be easily woken. A catnap is considered stage 1 type sleep.

We then cycle into stage 2. This is also a light stage but brain wave frequency increases. Eventually, brain waves slow down. If you decide to take a power nap, you'd be better served to wake up after cycling through stage 2, otherwise you'll feel groggy when you awaken. This means your power nap should be no longer than approximately 20 to 30 minutes in length.

Stages 3 and 4 are deep sleep cycles. During these stages, the brain produces slower delta waves. There is no eye movement or muscle activity. The body can repair muscles and tissues during this phase. Growth hormones are released, and development of the body and brain occurs. Immune function is supported and boosted through the buildup and storage of energy for the next day. During this stage of sleep, it is difficult to wake up. Our body becomes less responsive to the outside world. These stages of sleep are extremely restorative to the body.

After 90 minutes of entering stage 4, Rapid Eye Movement (REM) occurs. There are many cycles within REM. Each can last up to an hour. On average, most of us have about five or six REM cycles per night. During REM, our brain becomes highly active. This is the time when dreams occur. Breathing quickens, becoming fast and shallow, and eye movement increases, thus the name. Heart rate and blood pressure also increase. REM is important because it plays a significant role in learning and memory function. We consolidate all of the information absorbed throughout the day, then process it and store it away.

WHEN AND HOW LONG?

The actual time of the night that you sleep does make a significant difference in the quality and structure of it. You consistently cycle through a series of 90-minute sleep cycles throughout the night. What changes is the ratio of time spent in non-rapid eye movement (nonREM) sleep and in REM sleep. Earlier in the night, between 9:00 PM and 12:00 AM, we spend more time in non-REM sleep than REM sleep. During the last few cycles of sleep, into the early morning, we spend much more time in REM. Regardless of when you fall asleep, people tend to spend more time in non-REM sleep. Research has suggested that non-REM sleep is deeper and more restorative than lighter, dream-infused REM sleep.

If you are a typical night owl, overall, you'll get more REM sleep than people who go to bed earlier. So, if you tend to get to bed at midnight, your sleep will be composed of lighter, REM-predominant sleep. Unfortunately, the reduction in deep, restorative sleep may leave you groggy and unrefreshed the next day. Additionally, the immune system and the body loses healing and reparation time. This can affect hormone creation and growth. It can also significantly impact your ability to heal quickly. Overall, your hormonal balance and energy levels throughout the day will not be optimal.

In a number of studies, it has been found that shift workers who work odd hours of the night have increased rates of obesity, heart attacks, earlier death rate and decreased brain efficiency. A significant decline in cognitive abilities has been shown to accumulate with increased amounts of shift work.

The length of time you sleep is also important, and the effects of shortened sleep have been shown to increase heart rate throughout the day. It's worth realizing, though, that the length of time spent sleeping is not necessarily the only critical factor in all this. It's just as critical to go to bed earlier at night. The body and the brain have a circadian rhythm, which has been set for hundreds of thousands of years. This circadian rhythm is an internal 24-hour clock that informs when you sleep, wake and feel hungry. The hypothalamus part of the brain controls your circadian rhythm. External factors such as lightness and darkness impact it. This is the reason your circadian rhythm coincides so strongly with the sunrise and sunset. When it's dark at night, your eyes signal the brain that it's time to sleep. The brain releases melatonin which is one of the hormones that make you feel tired. Melatonin has been found not only in the pineal gland in the brain, but also in a number of other organs throughout the body. In fact, melatonin has been found in large quantities in the gut and may serve to decrease stomach ulcer formation and improve gut health. It also has a positive effect on the little valve between the stomach and the esophagus, and improves gastroesophageal reflux or heartburn symptoms. Often people who suffer from heartburn or GERD have poor sleep and this can be helped with melatonin.

Ultimately, when it comes to the ideal bedtime, there is a window of opportunity between the hours of 8:00 PM and midnight. Getting to sleep between these hours allows your body to get the right amount of non-REM and REM sleep needed for optimal health. The time you choose to go to bed within that window is somewhat influenced by your genetics. Some people prefer earlier and others prefer later. Listen to your body and the signals it is giving you about the sleep it needs each night. This will likely fluctuate a bit depending on how much rest you need at the moment. Additionally, as you age, your ideal bedtime will also change. It's been shown to be beneficial to keep your rising time in the morning to approximately the same each day within an hour or so. This is less likely to disrupt your circadian rhythm and reinforces the ability to sleep quickly at bedtime.

To summarize, the length of time you sleep is not necessarily your only concern. It's just as critical to go to bed between 8:00 PM and 12:00 AM at night, and wake up around the same time every morning.

TO NAP OR NOT?

Let's turn our attention to napping. In Western society, we tend to sleep in one big chunk, typically at night, after 10:00 PM. Research has shown there may be some benefits to sleeping twice during the day, as the Spaniards and Greeks do. That may mean adding a nap or a siesta into your schedule, if you can. Sleeping during the day has been a part of many cultures throughout the Mediterranean for centuries. Many elements of the Mediterranean lifestyle, as noted in

The Blue Zones book by Dan Buettner, contribute to longevity. Sleeping twice a day may actually fit our circadian rhythms (a healthy sleep-wake cycle) a bit more closely than not. Taking a catnap or siesta may just be what you need to improve your overall energy. Many people naturally experience a mid-afternoon energy drop between 1:00 PM and 3:00 PM. Many times, the increased sleepiness can also be due to a high carbohydrate or sugar-filled lunch. If your lunch is typically a balanced one of protein and vegetables, and you still experience some sleepiness in the afternoon, try a short nap.

Alas, this may not be an option for people working a day job. If that's you, I recommend getting to bed earlier each night, and improving the quality of your sleep. And don't be dismayed. There are other ways to improve your circadian rhythm.

The body's circadian rhythm dictates sleep. Numerous factors can influence this rhythm and contribute to poor sleep including: increased exposure to screens during the day and late at night, LED and blue lights, and long work hours, to name just a few. Many people are out of sync with their natural sleep-wake cycle. This affects their ability to rest peacefully and recover from the stresses and strains put on their bodies and minds while awake.

SLEEP HYGIENE

By improving the external factors affecting your body's circadian clock, you will have deeper sleep, wake up more refreshed, and have better midday energy, which promotes mental clarity. Many people also report weight loss by getting back in sync with their natural circadian rhythm. Here are some ideas for how you can do just that:

1. Try lying with your head at least five feet away from any electric fields which include: electrical outlets, clock radios, phones, stereos, computers, TV screens and monitors. You can also cover screens with EMF-reducing fabric if you live in a studio apartment or small space where items cannot be moved.

2. Consider moving these devices outside of your bedroom, when feasible. We're still learning about the long-term effects of electromagnetic frequencies (EMFs) on the body. Research shows that increased exposure to EMFs, the pineal gland and production of melatonin and serotonin can be adversely affected.

Here are some further action steps I recommend to improve the quality of sleep and connect with your innate circadian rhythm.

1. Wake up and go to sleep at the same time every day. Ideally be asleep by 10:00 PM and wake up at 6:00 AM.

2. Don't exercise within two hours of bedtime.

3. Turn off all TVs, and cease screen time about one hour prior to bedtime.

4. Avoid watching the news in the evening. Taking a break from the news is good practice because news can be highly sensational and mostly negative. If you need to watch some news, try finding feel-good stories about people who've made a positive impact on the world.

5. If you need to be on your computer or phone, try a computer screen that blocks blue light. Blue light blocker glasses also work. Blue light suppresses

appropriate melatonin released in the brain, which is necessary for sleep. The glasses can be worn during the day as well as at night. There are many brands of blue light blockers. Here is one brand I like: http://bit.ly/truedarkglasses

6. Avoid full spectrum light after sunset. Use amber light bulbs or a salt lamp in your bedroom as a way to reconnect with your circadian clock. These are devoid of blue light. Turn these on in the morning when you wake up.

7. Get plenty of midday sunlight, as this helps increase serotonin and melatonin. Take a walk outside.

8. Don't drink caffeine after 3:00 PM.

9. Avoid eating large meals or spicy foods prior to bedtime. Finish your meal and all beverages, alcoholic and non-alcoholic, at least three hours prior to bedtime. Exception to this is a night-time herbal tea.

10. Limit computer use by scheduling email responses for the morning. Doing so can be stimulating and affect your ability to fall asleep.

11. Settle any conflicts you have prior to going to bed with those in your immediate vicinity.

12. Write down anything that's bothering you and put it away for the next day if you cannot settle any issue with someone in the evening.

13. Use essential oils such as lavender or chamomile to increase a sense of calm in your body. These oils can be diffused in the room or used in a bath prior to bedtime.

14. Sleep in a completely dark room. Use light-blocking window treatments as needed.

15. Start a relaxation practice at least 20 to 30 minutes prior to bedtime. This can consist of meditation, gentle yoga nidra, or drinking botanical teas such as chamomile or kava. If you choose teas, try to drink these earlier in the evening prior to 8:00 PM.

16. Try a guided visualization CD at bedtime such as: https://www.healthjourneys.com/audio-library/sleep-insomnia. You can also use this in case you wake up in the middle of the night.

17. Try the 4-7-8 breath method before bedtime or if you wake up in the night. Here is the practice:

    Although you can do the exercise in any position, sit with your back straight while learning the exercise. Place the tip of your tongue against the ridge of tissue just behind your upper front teeth, and keep it there through the entire exercise. You will be exhaling through your mouth around your tongue; try pursing your lips slightly if this seems awkward.

    • Exhale completely through your mouth, making a whoosh sound.

    • Close your mouth and inhale quietly through your nose to a mental count of four.

    • Hold your breath for a count of seven.

    • Exhale completely through your mouth, making a whoosh sound to a count of eight. This is one breath.

- Now inhale again and repeat the cycle three more times for a total of four breaths.

Note that you always inhale quietly through your nose and exhale audibly through your mouth. The tip of your tongue stays in position the whole time. Exhalation takes twice as long as inhalation. The absolute time you spend on each phase is not important; the ratio of 4:7:8 is important. If you have trouble holding your breath, speed the exercise up but keep to the ratio of 4:7:8 for the three phases. With practice, you can slow it all down and get used to inhaling and exhaling more and more deeply.

18. Keep a notepad by your bed, and jot down any ideas, concerns or worries that ruminate in your mind. This allows you to release them and if need be return to the issues clearheaded in the morning.

19. If you cannot sleep, try some relaxing herbal tea again, such as chamomile or kava.

Meditate for five minutes then lie down once your mind is calm.

20. If you take melatonin before bed, do so approximately 20 to 30 minutes prior to when you want to fall asleep.

RESOURCES

1. Guided visualizations: This audio can be listened to at bedtime or even when you awaken in the middle of the night.

   **https://www.healthjourneys.com/audio-library/
   sleep-insomnia**

2. Night-time and relaxing teas: Try this tea at night prior to bedtime.

   **http://www.traditionalmedicinals.com/products/
   nighty-night-valarian**

3. Blue light blocker glasses: Try wearing these glasses during the day and/or at night to improve melatonin production for healthy sleep.

   http://bit.ly/truedarkglasses

3

MOVE NATURALLY

"If we could give every individual the right amount of
nourishment and exercise, not too little and not too much,
we would have found the safest way to health."

-HIPPOCRATES

One of the most basic aspects that make us human is the ability
to walk on two legs. Evolution shows us that we were once
four-legged creatures who then stood up. Since the Industrial
Revolution and especially in the past 50 years, we have become
a species that now predominantly sits rather than stands
throughout most of the day. Sitting has created an unhealthy
lifestyle, which has drastically affected our health. The rate
of obesity is skyrocketing as are diabetes and cardiovascular
disease and our lack of movement is one contributor to these
conditions increasing.

The World Health Organization gives us a glimpse into
how the obesity epidemic has overtaken a large chunk of
humanity. In the mid-90s, there were an estimated 200 million
adults, and 18 million children under the age of five who were
obese. By 2000, the number of obese adults increased to

300 million. What's even more shocking is that this is a worldwide phenomenon. About one third of all Americans are classified as obese. Obesity is an underlying cause in cardiovascular disease, diabetes, and cancer. These conditions are among the top ten causes of death in America.

It's not that surprising to see increased rates of disease, as most of us are sitting in front of computers or TV sets while stuffing our faces with fast food and other unhealthy processed edibles detrimental to our well-being. We must take back our natural movement. If we don't, our species will continue to deteriorate resulting in shorter and shorter lifespans.

REASONS TO EXERCISE

Exercising naturally throughout the day is one way to combat the long hours of sitting while working. Natural exercise consists of walking, climbing, dancing, hopping, lifting or otherwise moving in a way that is consistent with your day-to-day activities. You don't actually need to set aside one hour a day to go to the gym, or a yoga class, or engage in some other workout routine. Regimes such as crossfit, running marathons and triathlons are great for increasing endorphin levels and achievement; however, most people do not need to take on these activities in order to reap the health benefits of exercise. You can improve your health greatly from simply adding more steps in to your day. For example, you can choose to climb the stairs instead of taking the elevator and you will still get the benefits of exercise. During a long work day, take quick breaks to walk briskly back and forth in your office or do a few jumping jacks to get the blood flowing and improve your brain focus and attention. These short bursts of movement throughout the day add up. And let's face it, it's easier to add these into your day than try setting aside a long block of time for exercise.

Consider what's getting in the way of you exercising and moving naturally on a daily basis. Is it a lack of time? Or do you find it boring? Maybe you're not motivated to get up from your chair because you don't feel the need to increase movement? Some argue that they are already thin, and don't need exercise to change their appearance. In such cases, I suggest looking at the term **skinny fat**. It's used to describe people who appear to be thin externally, yet have a lot of extra fat surrounding many of their major organs. Unfortunately, skinny fat people are at risk for diabetes and cardiovascular disease as well as cancer. Your appearance alone should not and cannot be the sole motivator for movement and exercise.

How can you find out if there is unnecessary fat surrounding your organs? This can be measured by various instruments that look at body composition or fat-to-muscle ratios. You might find these instruments at your local health fair or at a gym or spa. They can consist of caliper measurements or other modalities. You can also ask your doctor to refer you for a dualenergy x-ray absorptiometry (DXA) scan, which is done typically at a research lab or university exercise lab. This scan uses x-ray technology to provide estimates of fat, bone and muscle mass in the entire body and in specific areas of the body.

BENEFITS BEYOND BODY WEIGHT

The benefits of movement and exercise are not just fat loss or increase in muscle tone. There are many bodily processes that benefit as well, including detoxification, digestion, building healthy bones, and improving brain concentration and attention. Research shows that strength training may lower a woman's risk for type 2 diabetes and cardiovascular disease.

Movements such as sitting up and down in a chair, jumping and lifting small boxes or cans overhead are also considered strength training. Using your own body weight to hold poses like plank, or do a few reps of push-ups or squats at short intervals throughout the day can be an effective way to build strength.

Movement and exercise also decreases the inflammatory response in the body and helps improve such conditions as cardiovascular disease and diabetes. We see improved insulin resistance, blood sugar control, and decreased cholesterol with regular exercise.

As we age, our bones become weaker if we maintain a sedentary lifestyle. Bones are constantly remodeling themselves. Bearing weight on your bones stresses the bones in a good way so that they rebuild stronger. The stronger your bones and muscles, the less fatigued you will feel from doing your day-to-day activities. You will be able to carry your groceries up the stairs, chase your kids around the yard and pick up heavy items in our home with ease.

Movement helps us to express the many different genes that we have. For example, a number of studies have shown that after engaging in any type of exercise, the genes that are linked to reducing inflammation and stress in the body are activated. This activation occurs whether you are simply taking a brisk walk around the block, or lifting weights at the gym. So, if getting to a gym is not something you enjoy or can fit into your life, rest assured that you can influence your genes in a positive way by engaging in short bursts of activity throughout your day.

Moving naturally also plays a big role in how we feel. Countless studies going back as far as the 1980s show the link between exercise, mental health and mood. They consistently prove that walking just 30 minutes a day is as effective, or more beneficial, than taking an antidepressant medication. That's incredible! That's what Mother Nature has given us: a free and natural tool to combat anxiety and depression, our legs. In fact, if these conditions of anxiety or depression are diagnosed, exercise should be given as the first prescription to combat those debilitating mental health issues. Your physician's toolbox now includes your legs as a treatment option.

Want a natural stress buster? Exercise can lower your stress and help you get your calm on. It does so by acting on the hypothalamic-pituitary-adrenal (HPA) axis, which engages your nervous system to help you relax. Acute stress causes excess hormones to be released from the adrenals, which then activates the sympathetic nervous system. Over time, this prolonged stress can cause a decrease or a deficiency in the same hormones, which then leads to several conditions of ill health including chronic fatigue, weight gain, and decreased libido. Regular aerobic exercise lowers the sympathetic nervous system and balances the HPA axis. Your hormone production normalizes and symptoms of stress disappear. In addition, the HPA axis plays an important role in the development of anxiety and depressive symptoms. It actively creates symptoms of fatigue and chronic fatigue. Therefore, supporting these organs and their functions through regular engagement in movement and exercise results in a better mood, a body that feels good and an optimized mind.

4

WHERE THE MIND GOES,
THE BODY FOLLOWS

"We must learn to reawaken and
keep ourselves awake."

~ HENRY DAVID THOREAU

You may have experienced pulling in to the parking lot at your child's school, but having no recollection of driving there. You may also have realized in mid-conversation that you can't recall what you were just talking about. You feel frustrated. Or perhaps you read and reread a paragraph and can't focus on the meaning of the story. These are symptoms of a distracted mind. Your mind has been rehashing the argument you had with your child before dropping him off at school. Or perhaps it's hanging out in the future, fretting the upcoming talk you have to give in front of a large audience. When you bring your awareness back to your physical sense, you realize that your heart rate is increased, your breath has quickened and you are starting to feel a pit in your stomach signaling anxiety. Your distracted mind caused you to miss the moment and the experience of what was actually happening in the present. A meandering mind can lead to depression, anxiety and ruminating thoughts. This can further lead to chronic psychological and physical stress as the mind continues on its negative pathways. Over time, the pattern of thoughts about the past, or projections about the future are repeated and a stress reaction in the body happens multiple times in a day. Symptoms such as fatigue, psoriasis, headaches and numerous other ailments manifest as a result of the chronic stress and inflammation caused by the untamed mind leading the body towards this fate. So, how do you tame the mind to not be lead astray by thoughts that aren't serving you in the present moment? The opposite of the meandering or wandering mind is a mindful one.

Finding ways to incorporate mindful practices into your life will allow you to retrain the nervous system. If we are always in a mode of reacting to our environment through unconscious triggers without even a second's pause to consider an alternative, we begin to wear ourselves out. Our sleep becomes non-restful, our digestive system becomes unbalanced, and ultimately, we begin to feel depleted and tired. By giving our brains a chance to rest, we can interrupt the stress response in the body which has become automatic and out of our conscious control. So, how do we rest our brains?

The good news is that the science of mindful practices is new, but the methods are old. You can teach an old dog new tricks. When I was in medical school, our understanding of the brain was that it stopped developing by the time you were 18 years old. In early childhood, there is an intense amount of growth and reorganization that happens in spurts. However, as it turns out, these processes continue on through our adulthood even until the last day of life. Two decades ago, I was taught that we only utilize a tiny percentage of our brain, and much of how we use it is predetermined based on our genetics and early childhood experiences. Our understanding of what the brain is capable of and its ability to change or remain static has completely shifted from those outdated ideas. This is largely due to improved technology, which allows us to look at brain anatomy and function in real time. We can observe areas of the brain that light up during particular tasks or activities, as well as measure brain growth over time. Our paradigm has shifted away from the belief that we cannot change and grow the brain to the now widely accepted understanding of neuroplasticity. Brain neuroplasticity refers to the brain's capacity to recover, reorganize and restructure itself. How it does so is based on the principle that "neurons that fire together wire together."

WIRING TOGETHER

Let's explore this concept in simple terms. The brain is made up of neurons. These neurons are like telephone cables carrying messages from one place to another. The place where two neurons meet is called a synapse. The synapse is a small gap where neurotransmitters or brain chemicals are released from one neuron to the other to continue passing on the message. When particular neurons are fired and the messages are passed down those lines, they get stronger. So, for example, if you happened to get stung by a bee as a child, it likely created a stress response in your body which engaged your sympathetic nervous system and caused your body to experience pain, an increased heart rate, increased blood pressure, and maybe even resulted in crying or screaming. The pathway in your brain that activated was the pain response. These neurons fired up and told your body that something dangerous happened so you had better take notice! Your brain also connected the experience to the bee, so in the future, whenever you see a bee, your brain automatically is triggered by the fear of pain and a stress response in your body occurs. These neurons wire together and fire together.

Traumatic experiences are not the only factor that influence how the brain is wired. Repetitive behavior, your environment, and chronic inner chatter also cause a change in neural pathways and synapses. In addition to strengthening particular pathways, the brain can also delete connections that are no longer useful or necessary.

An opportunity arises to retrain the brain and one of the most effective ways to do so is to engage in practices of focused awareness. There are many methods for practicing focused awareness, but one of the most well-studied is that of mindfulness meditation.

MINDFUL PRACTICES

Mindfulness meditation is originally a Buddhist technique that has evolved into various courses and practices over the years. The focus of mindfulness is to notice when we depart from the experience of the present moment and then choose to return. It is having awareness of feelings and thoughts as they come and go but not attaching to them. In the United States, clinical application of Mindfulness meditation began in the 1970's and the research has advanced as brain imaging technology has emerged. We are now able to map how this powerful ancient technique can change the manner in which different parts of the brain communicate and how this influences thought and creates lasting change in behavior. We have evidence that this practice helps with everything from anxiety and depression to chronic pain, addiction, irritable bowel syndrome and cancer.

Here is what happens to your mind after an eight-week practice of mindfulness:

The amygdala, which is the part of the brain involved with the "fight or flight" response, shrinks. The amygdala is the seat of fear and emotion and initiates a stress response. It is primal and old. The pre-frontal cortex, associated with higher level thinking, concentration and decision-making grows. These changes in the brain can be seen on MRI.

The connection between these regions of the brain is also altered. The connection between the amygdala and the rest of the brain weakens. The connections in the pre-frontal cortex strengthen. This causes a reduction in various chemicals in the body that are associated with stress and inflammation, such as cortisol, interleukin-6, and C-reactive protein. These changes in the brain were also associated with how people actually felt. Their psychological well-being improved. A study done at Johns Hopkins looked at mindfulness meditation and its ability to reduce symptoms of pain, depression and anxiety. They found that the effect of meditation on these symptoms was equivalent to the effect of antidepressants on these same symptoms.

Basic Mindfulness Meditation

Incredibly, just a few days of training leads to the benefits of mindfulness meditation.

Here is a basic practice to get started:

Step 1: Set aside dedicated meditation time. You don't need a meditation cushion or a studio, or any sort of unique equipment to access your mindfulness skills— however you do need to set aside a time and place for the practice.

Step 2: Sit comfortably. Find a place that gives you a stable, comfortable seat. Initially, if you need to lie down, do so. If on a cushion, cross your legs comfortably in front of you. If on a chair, rest the bottoms of your feet on the floor. Straighten your upper body and back without stiffening. Gently rest the palms of your hands on your legs, palms face up. If that doesn't feel natural, find a natural resting place for your arms and hands.

Step 3: Soften your gaze. Drop your chin a little and let your gaze fall gently downward. You can close your eyes or leave them open slightly. If your eyes are open slightly, let your vision soften so that you are not focusing on anything in particular.

Step 4: Begin to feel your breath. Bring your attention to the physical sensation of breathing. Feel the air move in through your nose or mouth. Feel the rise and fall of your chest initially, then your belly.

Step 5: Take notice of when your mind wanders away from your breath. When this happens, gently bring your attention back to the breath. It's typical for the mind to wander. It has been trained to do so for many years. The aim of mindfulness is not to stop the creation of thought or to quiet the mind. It a simple goal of paying attention to the present moment without judgement.

There is no need to work at blocking or clearing those thoughts and no need to worry that your mind wanders many times in a second. The mind is used to judging our thoughts, environment, prior actions and potential future. Let these thoughts arise without attaching a good or bad to them. Think of them as leaves on the river passing by. Make note of them and let them continue on their journey.

Even the most advanced practitioners have been through this and continue to have this experience depending on the day. Over time, you will notice less mind wandering with practice.

Step 6: Treat your wandering mind with kindness. Instead of wrestling with your thoughts, practice observing them without reacting. Treat your wandering mind as gently as you would a child. Initially, every time you bring your mind back to your breath, you might say "welcome home". As hard as it is to maintain, that's all there is. Come back to your breath over and over again, without judgment or expectation.

This is an example of a mindfulness practice. It may seem difficult or simple depending on the day. The goal is to just do the work. The results will happen. There are many mindful practices that you can begin to explore such as mindful walking and mindful eating. Each of these practices strengthens our attention and focus and allows the body to free itself from a reactive state, thereby improving energy and vitality.

Besides mindful practices, there are other forms of meditation that are just as effective at achieving the same results. I urge you to try them out. You can start with a commitment to five or ten minutes a day. You can use tools like apps for your phone such as Headspace: **https://www.headspace.com/headspace-meditation-app** or Insight Timer: **https://insighttimer.com/**

Heart-Centered Meditation

Another meditation I love is called the Heart-Centered Meditation. This particular meditation helps us shift from our head into our heart and alters our experience of our body and the world around us. The heart center has a tremendous healing energy. I learned this practice from my teacher and mentor, Dr. Anne Marie Chiasson, who is the co-director of the fellowship at the Arizona Center for Integrative Medicine. She learned this practice from her teacher.

This practice can be done daily for five to twenty minutes at a time. It is meant to allow for movement should you feel the desire to move.

> **Step 1:** Sit in a comfortable position and place your hands in the heart-center hand position. The heart center is found at the center of your breastbone in the center of your chest. You can lay one had over the other with the left hand lying on the chest and the right hand on top of the left hand.
>
> Exert a very slight pressure, just so that you feel the hands on the heart center.
>
> **Step 2:** Close your eyes, and with each breath, silently repeat the heart center attributes as a sacred prayer. The attributes of the heart center are:
>
> Compassion
> Innate harmony
> Healing presence
> Unconditional love

You can move through them in succession with each breath, or repeat one attribute 5-10 times, then the next, then the next. Try to embody each attribute and feel the infinite quality of it. If you feel the need to move or sway gently, you can do so.

Metta Meditation: The Meditation of Forgiveness

Metta is the practice of loving kindness. This exercise is a wonderful practice to shift energy in the body towards forgiveness of a specific person, situation or yourself. When you do this meditation, keep the words near you in the beginning so that you can read them. Once you know the meditation by heart, you can close your eyes while doing it. This meditation can be done daily.

Step 1: Sit in a comfortable position with your feet resting on the floor or cross-legged. Place your hands on you lap gently, palms facing upwards.

Step 2: Think of someone you love, and someone you are having difficulty with. The meditation will include these beings.

Step 3: Begin to slow your breath and focus on the words in front of you.

Step 4: Repeat all four of the following stanzas, four times each:

May I be at peace, may my heart remain open, may I awaken to the light of my own true nature, may I be healed, may I be a source of healing for all beings.

Bring up someone you love.

May you be at peace, may your heart remain open, may you awaken to the light of your own true nature, may you be healed, may you be a source of healing for all beings.

Bring up someone you have difficulty with.

May you be at peace, may your heart remain open, may you awaken to the light of your own true nature, may you be healed, may you be a source of healing for all beings.

Choose a group, family or all living things.

May we be at peace, may our hearts remain open, may we awaken to the light of our own true nature, may we be healed, may we be a source of healing for all beings.

There are numerous ways to engage in mind-body practices. These include breathwork such as the 4-7-8 breath, biofeedback techniques, guided visualization, self-hypnosis, and many more. I choose to focus on meditation as it is one of the areas in which we have mounting scientific evidence on its ability to change the wiring of the brain as well as the structure of it. Choose whatever suits you and your lifestyle, just choose to commit to something. Implement your chosen practice into your routine, until it becomes a habit and part of your day as is brushing your teeth. The health of your brain also requires constant attention, nourishment and commitment. The body will respond to the positive changes in brain function, the same way the brain responds to the body.

5

CLEAN UP YOUR ENVIRONMENT

"Keep close to Nature's heart... and break clear away, once in a while, and climb a mountain or spend a week in the woods. Wash your spirit clean."

~ JOHN MUIR

Most common diseases are caused by an interplay of your environment and the genes you were born with. You may be aware of the impact that chemicals in your food, pollutants in the air and heavy metals in your water have on your health. However, did you know that there are other more subtle exposures you have in your day to day life that affect the way your genes behave? These include things like electromagnetic frequency (EMF) from your technology, Bisphenol A that accumulates on your hands when you touch a restaurant receipt and even formaldehyde that seeps into the air from your new furniture. There are over 120 million industrial chemicals that have been registered and none of them have been tested adequately to evaluate what effects they have on our complex human being. Our bodies were not designed to be burdened by all these chemicals. The average woman puts over 150 synthetic chemicals on her body every day, none of which have been tested to see how they interact with her genes or her microbiome. In fact, even newborn babies are now found to have chemicals in their blood at birth. In a study spearheaded by the Environmental Working Group, they found that umbilical cord blood had over 287 synthetic chemicals found in it at birth. Of those, 180 of the chemicals are known to cause cancer in humans and animals and 217 are known to be toxic to the developing brain and nervous system of infants.

The interplay between our genetic makeup and the environmental exposure that we have throughout our lifetime can be complex. So much depends on what the makeup of your genes and your microbiome are, how these chemicals interact with each other in your body, how well you are able to detox these chemicals out of your body and how much fat tissue, which stores many of these chemicals, you have on your body. There are studies underway that will help us understand how the thousands of chemicals we inhale, ingest and absorb are affecting our longterm health. In the meantime, however, there are a few things we do know right now that can help us minimize our environment causing harm to our health.

Specifically, there are substances in the environment known as *endocrine disruptors* that have a similar chemical structure as our body's natural hormones. They can be natural or manmade. When they are absorbed into the body, they can interfere with the normal hormonal system. Research has found links between exposure to these chemicals and a woman's risk of breast cancer as well as other conditions such as diabetes and autoimmune disease. We also know that during particular phases of development, such as in-utero, early childhood and puberty, the opportunity for endocrine disruptors to wreak havoc on the hormonal system is at its greatest. All in all, it is best to avoid exposure to these substances. But how can we do that when we encounter these chemicals in such commonly used items as plastic toys, canned foods, personal care items, furniture, and electronics, and even in contaminated air, water and house dust?

What can be done to limit exposure?

- Eat hormone-free meat and dairy

- Reduce consumption of animal fat

- Use the Dirty Dozen list when deciding which fruits and vegetables to buy organic

- Use a water filter that removes chemicals, heavy metals and infectious agents

- Use stainless steel or glass containers

- Use only glass or ceramic (not plastic) in the microwave

- Eliminate phthalate-containing (PVC plastic) household items, toys, and personal care items

- Eliminate products containing "fragrance"

- Use non-toxic cleaning products

- Avoid chemical-based dry cleaning

- Avoid car exhaust and gasoline fumes

- Consider a HEPA filter to improve your indoor air quality

- Dust and vacuum your home frequently

- Consider adding plants to your home that help remove specific toxins. Here's a link to a list of those plants:

  http://www.cnn.com/2016/09/14/health/toxic-chemicals-housedust/index.html

Finding reputable online resources to research products can be confusing. I like to refer to the Environmental Working Group as a quick guide for many things such as the invaluable Dirty Dozen list: **http://www.ewg.org**

RESOURCES

In addition, you can use the below resources to research particular chemicals found in your products. Information is key. It can help you make healthier choices for yourself and your family, as well as giving you the tools to encourage industry and companies to improve their current practices.

1. Household Hazardous Substances Database links over 6,000 consumer brands to health effects.

   https://hpd.nlm.nih.gov

2. Agency for Toxic Substances Disease Registry (ATSDR) evaluates the human health effects of hazardous substances.

   http://www.atsdr.cdc.gov

3. The National Institute for Occupational Safety and Health (NIOSH) provides information on chemical safety, workplace health hazard evaluations and information regarding reproductive health.

   http://www.cdc.gov/niosh

Chemicals are not the only toxic factor infiltrating your home and affecting your health. Take a break from environmental noise and calm your mind. There is often much distressing world news. When you hear about these disturbing events, you might find that your stress response activates and you become reactive. You might feel powerless, sad and fearful at times. Now is the time, more than ever before, to focus on keeping a calm mind. By doing so, you can continue to act from a place of love, peace and security instead of from a place of fear.

Stress is anything that upsets our mind and body's equilibrium. Certainly, listening to the global reports of violence and tragedy qualifies as stress. The stress response is an automatic response in the body and triggers a series of inflammatory changes. The sympathetic nervous system is activated and a stream of hormones such as cortisol and adrenaline is released. Your heart beats faster, your muscles tighten, your blood pressure rises, and you become alert and tense. When this happens multiple times over and over again, it is difficult for your body and mind to settle down. Getting stuck in this "on" position can cause long-term changes to your neurons and immune system, leading to chronic conditions like hypertension, cardiovascular disease, chronic fatigue, autoimmune disease and an upset in our mental health. There is not much you or I can do about the news on TV (other than turn it off); however, you can help support and strengthen your body's ability to become more resilient and remain calm.

There are, of course, mind-body practices such as mindfulness meditation that you can do to reduce the stress response. These are discussed in the chapter on mind-body practices. Most importantly, though, be sure to take breaks from the news, social media and sensational events that don't promote feelings of well-being.

6

CULTIVATE THE RIGHT MINDSET FOR SUCCESS

"Keep your thoughts positive because your thoughts become your words. Keep your words positive because your words become your behavior. Keep your behavior positive because your behavior becomes your habits. Keep your habits positive because your habits become your values. Keep your values positive because your values become your destiny."

– MAHATMA GANDHI

So far, so much information. The truth is you can have all the best information in the world, listen to the stories of others and even take their advice, but if you don't *believe* that you deserve to thrive, you won't see your life improve. This is because you are either playing the role of martyr or victim, so as a result, your mindset won't allow you to implement anything that might help you heal and get better in the long run. Simply put, you don't buy into the idea that things can be different.

In order for all of this to work and for you to make real sustainable changes in your life, you must believe that you are worth it. You also must believe that you can change. You are surrounded by a lot of noise in a culture that tells you that you cannot change and at the same time pushes you to just "get over it" immediately without the discipline to feel your true emotions, let alone process them. Let me paint a picture. As an example, you are bombarded with fast food commercials and restaurant meals laden with bad oils, sugar, salt and hidden ingredients in your food. You didn't ask for this. You didn't ask for toxic fertilizers and neuroendocrine disruptors in your food. All of this was happening around you as we became a culture of convenience and quick fixes. You bought into the convenience of all that, as did the rest of us. Who doesn't appreciate the easy-to-hold food options available at the 7-Eleven down the street from work that you can grab and eat on the way back to your office desk?

Unfortunately, though, convenience has crippled us. The unintended side effects of offering ease and efficiency has left us with insulin resistance, obesity, and hormonal imbalance. Foods that promised to be so wholesome and good, conveniently packaged in a box or can, offer none of that. What they offer is added harmful ingredients, a lack of nutrients and an unwanted addiction to the neurochemical ingredients found in the so-called food. This results in an imprisonment of your mind and your body.

Your body struggles to heal and restore itself. Without the foundational pieces, its energies are diverted towards figuring out how to attack the numerous chemicals that you've added into your bloodstream through hidden food additives. Your poor body is confused and disempowered. It cannot accomplish the tasks it needs to do because the foundation is shaky; yet it requires a solid base from which to grow. Without that solid base, the building blocks are not provided for the cells to work efficiently, create energy and participate in other metabolic processes.

Your body so desperately wants to move as it was intended to do. You have deadlines to meet and work to do and your work requires you to sit in front of the computer at a desk for hours on end. When given the choice to walk or drive, you choose to drive, so that you can save extra time. I get it. You are busy. And every minute counts.

This pattern of unnatural living continues. At night, your body starts sending the signals that it's time to sleep. Your melatonin levels start to go up and body temperature starts to drop. Digestion slows down. You begin to feel sleepy. However, you have one more email to answer, just a few more things to get done. The addictive reality TV show is grabbing your attention and hard to turn off. So you ignore the signals and just stay up a little bit longer pushing past the desire for sleep. Eventually, your body revolts by sending signals: "Enough is enough!" What signals do I mean? It starts with symptoms of fatigue and changes in hormones.

This might be followed by the inability to think as clearly as you once did. You might think these changes are happening simply because you are getting older. You are led to believe - falsely - that you are feeling this way because of your genetics. Your entire family has had thyroid disease or diabetes or hormonal imbalance and eventually you will too. That is what your friends, family and maybe even your doctor tells you. You think that this is just the way it's supposed to be because everyone else around you is feeling the same way. Everyone else is eating the same food. They're going to the same restaurants and they're working and they're managing their life just like you are. Did you ever wonder if it could be different? Did you ever think that it's not the way things have to be?

Maybe you use your physical condition as a badge of honor. Or maybe you feel that you are tired and overweight and ill because you work hard and keep busy. Because aren't these just the consequences of hard work and busy-ness? You lead a full life and you get a lot of stuff done. Isn't it the side effect of those choices?

I know about all this not just because I'm a medical practitioner, but because I've lived that life as well. Like you, I struggled to get everything done to keep my home running, while raising my kids, and managing a successful career. I multi-tasked to save time (or so I thought) and to be more efficient. I thought I was Superwoman. Yet it came with a high price tag.

I was so busy with work that I wasn't even able to relax on vacation. From the moment I arose, I was on the go and didn't stop until it was time to lay my head down on the pillow. I didn't allow my body even a few seconds of rest during the day. My nervous system didn't have a chance to calm down. My body was simply fulfilling the demands that I put on it until it no longer could.

I'm here to tell you that things don't have to manifest that way. You can be efficient, accomplish all of your goals, and still take care of your body, mind and soul. Doing so requires a shift in your mindset.

First, you have to know that *you are good enough* and that *you are loved*. You are deserving of a healthy and vibrant body and mind and spirit.

Second, you have to believe that being busy is not an excuse. You get to choose what occupies your time and attention, not the other way around. Don't let time and attention choose to occupy you.

Third, you are not controlled by your genetics. The choices you make on a day-to-day basis in your life determine whether or not those genes express themselves, so don't let any doctor or family member - or anyone for that matter - tell you that you'll get a particular disease because you have the gene for it. This is simply not true. In fact, only approximately 10% or fewer of your genes will result in disease no matter what you do. That means that 90% or more of your genes will express themselves based on the choices that you make in your life. This is empowerment! This affords you the opportunity to choose your destiny, not let your destiny choose you.

So, if your genes aren't responsible for disease, then what is? The *exposome* refers to all the non-genetic exposures you've had in your entire lifetime. This includes the food you eat, the water you drink, the social interactions you have, the air you breathe and even the health of your parents at the time of your conception. In sum, it is the full range of environmental exposures and lifestyle choices from birth to death that has a greater effect on your health than your genes. You can think of it like this: "Your genes load the gun, but the environment pulls the trigger."

Fourth, understand that you continue to think the way you do and make the choices you make because you are feeding your mind and body the same information that you have always given it. If you give yourself the same information, you will keep seeing the same results. You must believe that things can be different. You must envision a new healthier version of yourself. If you start with a desired version of yourself and project it outwardly, then you allow the internal environment to dictate who and what you are, rather than allowing the external environment to shape and mold you. This is, in my opinion, true freedom. To start, practice this exercise:

- First, write down three things that you want in your life. For example, increased energy, clear thinking, and movement without pain.

- Every morning when you wake up write down three sentences as if you already have these things in your life. The example here would read like this: *I have boundless energy to do the things I want every day. I have movement without pain and can walk for as long as I like pain-free. My mind is clear and my thoughts make sense.*

- Then spend a few minutes really honing in on the details of what that looks like. Envision yourself walking to the store without anything hurting. See yourself waking up in the morning and having so much energy that you are able to start your day with joy and end your day with full satisfaction that you were able to complete your list of goals for the day. Imagine all of the details. Envision yourself having clarity of thought and having fruitful conversations with people or finally writing that book you wanted to write because your brain is able to work so efficiently. The more you are able to imagine the details of what this feels like, the more successful you will be.

- Try to use all five senses. What does a morning full of energy **smell** like? What does your body **feel** like when it walks without pain? What are you **hearing** along your walk? How does the morning air **taste** along your walk? What do you **see** with your clear mind on your walk? Flesh out the details of this vision. Truly feel as though this reality already exists for you.

Remember, neurons that wire together fire together. This means that as your mind literally experiences the joy of a pain-free body, a clear mind and boundless energy, it begins to remodel itself. By envisioning the details of your experience, you fire up the brain cells and the pathways in the brain that are associated with that experience. Your brain feels as though it has already gone through the motions of having increased energy, clarity of mind, and a strong body without pain. Where the brain goes, the body follows. Once the brain begins to consciously mentally rehearse the new you, new circuits are activated in new ways to rewire a new mind. Then your thoughts create an experience, and via the emotional brain, new emotions are also produced. The body is then conditioned by the new mind and a new state of being is programmed into your subconscious. When you think of who you want to be versus who you no longer want to be, the old neural circuits in the brain begin to die off because you are not activating them. The old thought patterns that are not serving you are pruned away. You create new circuitry in the brain when you rehearse the new person that you want to be. This is a powerful method for creating new habits and a new you.

Follow this intention-setting exercise with a gratitude practice. This is as easy as writing down three things that you are grateful for at that moment. Here's an example:

I am grateful for being able to watch my son's soccer game.

I am grateful to be able to enjoy a peaceful walk on the lake.

I am grateful for being able to have eaten a nourishing meal last night.

A regular practice of gratitude simply means taking the time to notice and reflect upon what you are thankful for. Engaging in the practice frequently has been shown to increase positive emotions, enhance sleep, nurture compassion and kindness, and improve the immune response.

I suggest you start your day with this practice, because it gets your mind in the right framework and informs the rest of your day. Throughout the day, take notice and give thanks for everything you have in your life, the people who bring you joy and the experiences you are able to appreciate. Cultivate an attitude of gratitude.

These practices will get your mind and body in the right place so that when you begin to feed it good information by replenishing nutrients and correcting imbalances, both mind and body will respond positively. Removing blockages and providing support allows the communication between mind and body to flow freely. Your body will react as though it already knows what to do. It will respond because you have rehearsed the outcomes in your mind thousands of times. Your body will already know what it feels like to move pain-free, to have clarity of thought and to experience the joy of boundless energy.

The brain has already experienced these results through all five senses through your visualization practice and has rewired itself into a new pattern. This all begins with your mindset. You have to believe that you can change your body and your mind. You have to believe this in your core. And you have to believe that you deserve the life that you envision.

7

CONNECTION TO COMMUNITY IS YOUR ANTIDOTE TO LONLINESS

"When 'I' is replaced with 'we',
even illness becomes wellness."

~ MALCOLM X

We've talked a lot about how eating a well-balanced, plant-based diet can improve your health. We've explored how working out and moving naturally have benefits for health. We've reviewed sleep architecture and the necessity for restful sleep. We know all of these things improve our health outcomes, but did you also know that having social connection is just as critical to your health?

Humans are hard-wired to connect. As an example, you experience this connection when you are in conversation with someone. Your brain contains nerve cells called neurons that mirror the emotions of the person you are talking to. Your facial muscles also have similar movements. You feel empathy and similar emotions. There is a moment-to-moment resonance that connects you and the other person. If we were able to look at your brain, we would see that you and the person you are in conversation with are *lit up* in the same areas. You are literally connected and in coherence. There have been numerous studies that show loving relationships improve our health outcomes and can even decrease pain. From the time of your birth, your survival depends on social connection. When babies cry, mothers have a brain response that resembles pain. This ensures that the baby's needs for food, shelter and safety are met.

In fact, it has been shown that isolation and lack of human connection can be detrimental to your health. Studies have suggested that a lack of social connection can have a greater negative impact on your health than obesity, hypertension and smoking. Studies have also indicated that strong social connection can result in a 50% increased longevity, lower levels of anxiety and depression, faster recovery from disease, a stronger immune system, higher selfesteem and empathy for others.

Social isolation results in a decline in both mental and physical health, and increases the likelihood for antisocial behavior, which then leads to depression and further isolation. Sadly, social isolation is on the rise. Social isolation has doubled from 20% to 40% since the 1980s. This type of loneliness can increase the risk of heart disease by 29% and stroke by 32%. Despite these health detriments, over the last 50 years or so, social connections have been decreasing. Marriage rates are decreased, families are having fewer children, and many people report that they have fewer close friends than they would like. Not surprisingly, we are seeing higher rates of depression, suicide, drug addiction, chronic pain and unhappiness.

Loneliness also accelerates cognitive decline in older adults. This is the paradox of our hyper-connected digital age. We seem to be more connected through social media and online sources; however, we appear to be drifting apart and feeling more isolated. I oftentimes hear from patients in my clinical practice that it is difficult to make new friends, especially as we get busy with our lives. We are often running between dropping off the kids, work obligations, taking the kids to various activities, trying to manage the household…

Weekends used to consist of a day of rest and connection, especially on Sundays in America. But now? Most families are busy juggling sports or hobbies, catching up on the week, and sometimes just trying to catch their breath. Clearly, we've seen the benefits of remaining active and having friends are there, so how can we stay socially connected in our busy world?

Here are some ways to increase your social connection and improve health outcomes:

1. Practice gratitude by thanking one person each day. Gratitude is a two-way exchange.

   Not only will you make someone else happy, but your own happiness will also increase.

2. Engage in random acts of kindness. Kindness grows compassion. Increasing your feelings of compassion allows you to feel more connected with others and ultimately ups your own feel-good vibes.

3. Allow yourself to be vulnerable. Independence is considered a strength in our society. You may feel that opening up to others, showing your fears and worries or asking for support is a form of weakness. However,

doing so creates an opportunity for others to help, which increases social connection. Being vulnerable also allows us to deepen our existing relationships and eliminates feelings of social isolation. Most people appreciate the ability to connect on a deeper level.

4. Give mutual support to friends and family by practicing solidarity. Connecting on a singular purpose increases the closeness we feel with others.

5. Volunteer and give your time freely. Studies have shown that people who volunteer on a regular basis are happier than others. The act of altruism for the welfare of others keeps you connected to your community and even your purpose.

6. Engage in hospitality. An easy way to host friends and family is to cook a meal together and share the dinner table. Humans have hunted, gathered, cooked and eaten together for centuries. Continuing this evolutionary tradition improves our social interactions and brings us closer to others.

8

WHAT IS YOUR WHY? IDENTIFY SPIRIT AND PURPOSE

"The two most important days in life are
the day you born and the day you
discover the reason why."

– MARK TWAIN

It is important to define spirituality. I like the definition given by our former Surgeon General, Dr. C. Everett Koop, who defined spirituality as "the vital center of a person; that which is held sacred." I feel that this removes religion from the discussion, though many people define their spirituality in the context of religion. In truth, spirituality is much more than that, mostly because it is fluid, cannot be confined to a context, and will change with your personal experience. It is personal; unique to each individual. It is an experience first, and then words second. The spoken story of the experience of spirituality is the framework for how it is shared with others. It is manifested in all that we do, and influences our values, choices and behaviors.

This last attribute is the reason we find that connecting to your own spirituality and purpose affects your health outcomes.

Research shows that there is a connection between your beliefs and your well-being. Religion, prayer and meditation can provide comfort to people and a framework for how they might understand anything that feels out of their own control. Oftentimes, people gain strength and feel more positive through the practice of prayer or meditation. In fact, studies have shown that people who belong to a religious or spiritual community and attend activities regularly live an average of eight years longer. In one study, it was found that women who attended church more than once per week had a 33% lower risk of dying during the study period compared with those who reported that they did not attend church. Attending church even once per week was associated with a lower risk of death at 26% and attending less than weekly showed a decrease in risk of death by 13%.

Attending religious or spiritual services can offer social support and optimism, as well as lower rates of depression and smoking.

Positive beliefs, comfort and strength gained from religion, meditation, and prayer can contribute to well-being. These may even promote healing, help prevent chronic health problems and increase your resilience. Such practices, therefore, will allow you to cope better with illness, stress, or death. Committing to a spiritual or religious activity may not cure an illness, but it may help you *feel better*.

Figuring out your purpose may take a bit of introspection. When you do identify it, you will know, and this will drive you to do things in alignment with your perceived purpose. In fact, having a purpose for activities you choose to do will improve your brain function, increase happiness and lengthen your lifespan. In nursing homes, we see residents come alive again after years of non-communication when they are simply given a plant and tasked with keeping it alive.

A number of studies have demonstrated that having a purpose is linked to various health outcomes. These include a lower risk of dementia, decreased heart attacks and stroke, and improved sleep. Premature death and chronic disease resulting in disability are also lower in people who have found meaning in their lives. In fact, epigenetic changes have been seen, including decreased expression of genes that cause inflammation in the body.

Studies also show that people who have found a purpose for their life engage in more preventive health behaviors such as getting mammograms, colonoscopies and other screening tests. These tests have been shown to increase longevity and pick up early stage of disease where interventions are more likely to make a difference.

Here are some ways to cultivate spirituality and purpose:

1. Think about times in your life when you have had a sense of peace. Identify aspects of your life that bring you love, comfort, strength and hope.

2. Add prayer, meditation, singing or listening to devotional songs, reading inspirational books and getting out in nature to your daily routine.

9

IT'S ALL IN YOUR HEAD

"Love is old, love is new.
Love is all, love is you."

- THE BEATLES

As a doctor, I have seen with my own eyes how a person can heal their physical body. The body has an amazing capacity to heal itself. It works in tandem as a unified whole, connected to mind, emotions and spirit, through consciousness and energy. This energy is what connects us to others. It is what connects us to the greater power of healing.

In my two decades of seeing and treating patients, I often found myself asking the question: Why do some patients heal and others don't?

While I do not have the answer to this question, I do know that when we address what is at the core of our desires, what is deepest in our hearts and what is our biggest motivation for every choice we make in our lives, we open up to the possibility of healing.

So, what is at the root of our deepest desire? The answer is *love*. The desire to feel boundless, abundant, joyful love. This is the state of pure heart-centeredness. There are no blocks to this love, and it guides our intuition, empowers us and reminds us that we have the answers inside of ourselves. I am a doctor, but you are the healer. You are the one who can change the vibration of every single cell in your body by your thoughts and emotions alone. You might be wondering why this matters. And if it matters, you might ask: How *do* I access my heart center and open up the potential for healing?

First, you have to understand how the thought patterns in your brain cause a physical reaction in the body. Negative thoughts, scarcity mindset and living in fear are powerful drivers of ill health. The opposite is also true. Positive thoughts, abundance mindset and being at peace improves health outcomes. Let me explain further.

Have you had the experience of going to your doctor with concerns about feeling tired and maybe an increased heart rate, or feeling like your emotional state is a rollercoaster? Maybe you have digestive issues and a nervous stomach with bowel movements that alternate between constipation and diarrhea? After running a battery of tests and maybe even procedures, the doctor says to you a variation of the phrase: "It's all in your head." Well, hearing that was probably frustrating. It was not the answer you might have expected to hear. And while it's not *entirely* true, it's also not *entirely* false either. Perhaps the better answer from the doctor would have been: "It all started in your head."

Our thought patterns and emotions can influence our ability to heal. To explain how this happens, let's start with the nervous system. We each have one and this nervous system connects to every organ and influences every cell in our body.

Our nervous system can react in one of two ways. It either hangs out in a *parasympathetic* state where we are in a phase of resting and digesting. In this state, we heal and repair, as well as digest our food and absorb our nutrients. It's during this relaxation that our heart rates goes down and our blood pressure lowers. The body can send healing cells and signals throughout the body, wherever repair, healing and growth need to happen.

The other state our body can dwell in is *sympathetic*. This is also called the *fight-or-flight response*. During this state, our heart rate increases, blood pressure goes up, and blood is shunted away from the digestive system. The blood is sent to the muscles and they get *primed*. We are ready to respond to and react quickly to the threat or emergency in front of us. We experience an acute sense of fear if we are threatened physically, which is a survival mechanism; this reaction is meant to protect us. The flight-or-fight response activates with fear and allows us to move out of harm's way quickly.

Unfortunately for us, fear can also come from emotional thought patterns. Anxiety, worries about the future, fear about not being accepted and all the other imaginary projections we have can send us into a tailspin. The trouble is that the body can only respond one way. It cannot tell the difference between an emotionally driven fear and a physical fear or threat. Our adrenals kick on fast. We release adrenaline and cortisol, which triggers the same set of sympathetic responses (the increased heart rate, the blood pressure hike, and a number of others) in the body.

If worry, anxiety or fears are chronic, then the body is constantly bombarded with the stress response hormones and has barely any time to recover in the relaxation or parasympathetic state. Eventually, this flood of neurochemicals in the brain and hormones in the body will sensitize the brain to react even more violently to perceived threats whether emotional or physical. Our body records this new state of being as normal. After a time, we begin to feel chronically anxious with all the resulting physical symptoms occurring. You may not even remember what the initial trigger or threat was. Soon, the body takes over. It is simply doing what it is used to doing, and as a consequence, it becomes difficult to change course.

The body is so used to responding this way that even the smallest conscious or unconscious thought can put us into that body response. Oftentimes, it happens so quickly that you can't even stop it. This potent stress response not only affects your mind but also your body. Essentially, this survival mechanism, which was meant to be activated only in times of real physical threat, has now become your status quo. Your nervous system has been *hijacked*. No matter how hard you try to heal, you can't change the body's response because the information it is receiving is coming from unconscious processes in the mind. This is why I say it all starts in your head.

So how do we disrupt this powerful survival mechanism gone astray? The first step is in recognizing it; recognizing that the emotions, the fear, the anxiety, grief, and loss, as well as feelings of unworthiness, being unloved or unsafe, are the deep strong roots that tell the body how to react. Emotions are triggered one way or another, which affects how we eat, how we digest our food. Emotions also affect whether or not we are motivated to make change, whether or not we work out, and even how we sleep and dream.

CONCLUSION

Even though deep down I've always believed what I saw growing up that healing is defined not by fixing a problem with a pill, but through the spice blends and botanicals of my childhood, by eating mostly plants, through movement and rest, and from meditating for the good of the mind and the spirit, it was following the research that led us here to this book.

In chapter one, you saw how, while there is no single perfect diet for everyone, there are principles that you can follow to make sure you're getting the nutrition your body needs. And while your genetics, the state of your gut microbiome and other factors come into play, feeding your body essential nutrients and minimizing inflammation in the body is your aim. In fact, in order to put your body into as stress-free state as possible, a generalized anti-inflammatory diet is best for most people. The focus? Eating food with the minimal amount of processing and chemicals, being mindful of its source, and ensuring nutrients from vegetables are top priority.

Next, we focused on the importance of sleep, in particular learning about the impacts of disrupted sleep cycles and what to do about improving the sleep you get. Remember, it's not just about how much, but also when during the night you get that sleep. Using that knowledge of sleep, I also made plenty of suggestions for improving sleep quality, especially tips to try to improve relaxation in the evening and what to include in a bedtime routine.

In the following chapter, we covered the importance of including natural movement in this age where sedentary lifestyles are the norm. While incorporating some movement into your day is essential to thrive, not moving is common and comes with a long list of risks that we touched on in this chapter. Starting with walking, I recommended movement for improving health and busting stress, even if lack of exercise isn't showing up for you right now in your body weight.

Then we looked at how the brain wires and rewires through persistent thought patterns as well as the benefits of bringing awareness to a meandering mind. To avoid depression, anxiety and further psychological and physical stress, I outlined some mindfulness meditation techniques to give your brain a rest from its negative pathways. Encouraging you to stay in the present moment and notice when you depart from that experience, as well as having awareness of feelings and thoughts as they come and go but not attaching to them, I presented three main practices that you can use to forge your own mind-body connection: basic mindfulness meditation; heart-centered meditation; forgiveness meditation.

Chapter five was then packed with suggestions for reducing the hormone-disrupting toxins in your home environment, which is a frequently overlooked aspect to include in your plan to thriving health. And chapter six then looked at reading the signals, rather than believing everything you've ever been told about your health limitations; then kindly allowing yourself to believe you deserve a healthier, happier live, where you do indeed thrive.

Lastly, we turned our heads towards the loneliness epidemic and how humans are hardwired to connect with other humans, mirroring their emotions, feeling empathy and so on. Knowing how loving relationships improve your health, even decrease pain, and that isolation can be detrimental to your health, I offered a number of ways in which you can bring that allimportant social connection back into your life. Then in chapter eight, I encouraged finding that connection within yourself through a spiritual practice, and by doing so finding that social support and optimism, as well as harnessing positive beliefs, comfort and strength through meditation or prayer. That self-connection and connection to a higher being, no matter what your beliefs are, is said to even promote healing, help prevent chronic health problems and increase your resilience.

Built To Thrive has married the foundational pillars of health with the underlying science, helping you understand what's going on in your body and mind, and encouraging:

- well-balanced, plant-based nutrition

- working out and moving naturally

- restful sleep

- social connection

- mindful practices

- protection against and reduction of toxins in your environment

- belief that you can change.

Taking each of these principles individually has merit and can boost your health beyond mere survival. Yet to truly thrive requires that you follow through and make those improvements happen, even in tiny incremental steps, and to sustain them. Being built to thrive is not about making these changes for the short term or going on a diet for a few weeks or months. This is a lifestyle that will last a lifetime. And to work, you have to make it yours.

In my integrative medical practice, I talk about you feeling *empowered to make sustainable changes that fit your lifestyle and allow you to thrive.* That means you don't have to aim for perfect. Start exactly where you are right now. Experiment with some of the suggestions covered in this book. Set yourself up to succeed by looking at what you think can work and going from there. If you've read this far, you may already have a sense of what that first step is, so all that's left is to get started today. Because in reality, you have all you need available to you right now. You are ready and you are built to thrive.

If this book makes complete sense to you and you're in need of help right now, book a FREE discovery phone call here: https://BookwithDrSethi.as.me or FREE first appointment (in person) on my website here: https://www.drshellysethi.com

I would love to help you transform your health. Here's what you can expect from our first session:

When you come to the office, you will share your story and together we will review your lifestyle, including how you sleep, how you move, what you eat, your community and your relationships. We'll talk about how you may or may not be living your purpose and how you deal with stress. We also take a comprehensive look at labs that will give us more information about how your body is functioning on a cellular and physiological level.

Next, you will get a detailed plan and program taking you through the process of restoring your body to its natural healing capabilities. We'll review your results and recommend specific and personalized ways to help your body begin to heal and recover. We will optimize these processes on the cellular, energetic and spiritual and emotional level over the course of working together. I look forward to getting to know you.

Thank you for taking the time to read the information presented in this book. I hope you have found practical and usable tools that you have been able to implement right away. On the following pages, you will find a few of my favorite things: recipes and plant medicine. I have shared with you some of my favorite health-boosting recipes that I created and use in my own home. I have also included a beginner's guide to understanding the amazing healing benefits to the spices and herbs that I urge you to use on a daily basis. Enjoy!

FAVORITE RECIPES:

Curried Roasted Cauliflower Soup (serves 4)

Good time to serve:

I love this soup on a crisp fall day for dinner. It works well as a starter for a holiday dinner, such as at Thanksgiving.

Story behind this dish:

This is a blend of my ethnic heritage and my love for food as medicine. This recipe contains spices that have healing properties. The cauliflower, as a cruciferous vegetable, is a nutrientdense power food, which contains indoles (indole-3-carbinol) and flavones. These compounds have been shown to reduce breast, lung and colorectal cancer.

The garlic in this recipe contains allicin (released when exposed to air). Garlic lowers blood pressure, acts as blood thinner, is cardioprotective and fights infection. Additionally, the turmeric is a potent anti-inflammatory and used in cancer prevention. Turmeric decreases arthritic pain, and helps prevent Alzheimer's and inflammatory bowel disease.

Prep time: 15 minutes

Cook time: 45 minutes

Ingredients:

- *1 large head of cauliflower, broken into small florets, stems chopped*
- *5 tbsp extra virgin olive oil (organic, if possible)*
- *⅓ cup roasted unsalted cashews (or 1 cup of cashew milk)*
- *1 medium yellow onion, diced*
- *4 whole cloves of garlic*
- *14-ounce can of light coconut milk*

- *½ tsp ground coriander*
- *½ tsp ground turmeric*
- *1¼ tsp ground cumin*
- *¼ tsp ground cinnamon*
- *1 tsp cane sugar*
- *2 cups low sodium vegetable broth or water*
- *salt*
- *pepper*
- *¼ cup chopped cilantro*
- *¼ cup chopped chives*

Directions:

Preheat oven to 400°F. Toss the cauliflower and garlic cloves with enough olive oil to lightly coat it (about three tablespoons). Spread the cauliflower and garlic cloves in a single layer on a large baking sheet and roast until the tips of the cauliflower are golden brown, about 25 to 30 minutes.

Blend cashews in a blender until finely ground. Add ¾ cup of water and blend. Pour mixture through a fine-mesh strainer into a bowl and press on the solids with the spoon. Discard the solids. Alternatively, you can use ¾ to 1 cup of cashew milk.

In a Dutch oven or heavy pot, heat the remaining olive oil over low heat. Add the onions and sweat with a dash of salt. Continue cooking the onions until golden brown. Add the cauliflower, garlic, coconut milk, cashew milk, coriander, turmeric, cumin, cinnamon and sugar. Add the vegetable broth or water and simmer for 5 minutes.

Use an immersion blender to blend the soup to desired consistency. If using a blender instead of an immersion blender, allow soup to cool for 20 minutes and add to blender. Blend soup until it is smooth. Return to the pot and add salt and pepper to taste. Ladle into four bowls and top with chopped cilantro and chives.

Notes:

You can substitute the turmeric, coriander and cumin powder for two tablespoons curry powder.

To toast the cashews: Preheat the oven to 350°F and lay cashews out on a baking sheet in a nice flat layer. Toast for 5 to 6 minutes, or until fragrant.

Coconut Vegetable Soup with Cashew Cream

(serves 6-8)

Good time to serve:

This would be a great meal to serve with crusty bread on a cold winter day or even as an appetizer to your holiday meal.

Story behind this dish:

This dish was born out of my love of soups, turmeric and coconut. It is anti-inflammatory, full of healing spices and tasty.

Prep time: 30 minutes

Cook time: 30 minutes

Ingredients:

- *1 cup raw cashews, soaked*
- *6 cups organic vegetable or chicken broth*
- *2 tbsp extra virgin olive oil*
- *4 cloves of crushed garlic*
- *1 sweet or yellow onion, chopped*
- *3 medium carrots, chopped*
- *1½ cups peeled and chopped sweet potato, yam or butternut squash*
- *28-ounce can or jar diced tomatoes with juices*
- *2 stalks of celery, chopped*
- *2 tsp ground coriander*
- *2 tsp ground turmeric, fresh or powder*
- *¼ tsp black pepper*
- *1 tsp kosher salt*
- *2 bay leaves*
- *2 cups kale or chard, destemmed and torn*
- *15-ounce can chickpeas or other beans, drained and rinsed*
- *1 cup coconut milk or cream*
- *½ cup chopped cilantro*
- *squeezed juice of half a lime*

Directions:

In a blender, combine soaked and drained cashews with 1 cup of vegetable or chicken broth and blend until smooth. In a large saucepan, heat the olive oil over medium heat. Add the garlic and onions and sauté for 3 to 5 minutes until the onion is translucent.

Add the carrots, potatoes or squash, celery, diced tomatoes with juice, the remaining 5 cups of broth, the cashew cream and the coriander, and turmeric. Stir well to combine. Bring the mixture to a boil and then reduce the heat to medium-low. Season with salt and black pepper and add the bay leaves.

Simmer the soup, uncovered, for at least 20 minutes, until the vegetables are tender. During the last 10 minutes of cooking, add the chickpeas or beans, the Swiss chard or spinach, coconut milk or cream and lime juice.

Remove and discard the bay leaves before serving. Add the chopped cilantro prior to serving.

Notes:

This dish is versatile. You can add heat to it by adding paprika, cayenne or crushed red pepper. You can also use a variety of vegetables such as potatoes or other squashes.

Baked Spaghetti Squash (inspired by Dr. Andrew Weil) (serves 8)

Good time to serve:

This can be served anytime and could be a full meal with a green salad.

Story behind this dish:

This is the first dish I tried at Dr. Weil's True Food Kitchen and thought it was a delicious alternative to pasta. It's a wonderful way to introduce kids to healthy squashes as well.

- *Prep time: 20 minutes*
- *Cook time: 1 hour 30 minutes*
- *Ingredients:*
- *1 spaghetti squash*
- *2 large carrots, diced*
- *2 stalks celery, diced*
- *1 large yellow onion, diced*
- *1 red bell pepper, diced*
- *2 tbsp extra virgin olive oil*

- *1 large can (28 ounces) crushed tomatoes*
- *red pepper flakes*
- *1 tsp dried basil*
- *½ tsp dried oregano*
- *pinch of ground allspice*
- *3 cloves of chopped garlic*
- *¾ pound part-skim mozzarella*
- *½ cup grated Parmesan cheese*

Directions:

Place the spaghetti squash in a large pot of water (it should float) and bring to a boil. Lower heat, cover and boil gently for 50 minutes. Another option is to bake the squash first. Cut it lengthwise and place the halves skin-side down in a baking dish with an inch of water. Cover the dish with foil and bake at 350ºF for about 45 minutes, or until meat is tender. While squash is cooking, peel and slice the carrots, celery, onion and bell pepper.

Heat olive oil in a skillet and add the onion and carrot, with some water to prevent sticking. Sauté over medium heat for 5 minutes. Add remaining vegetables with some red pepper flakes and a dash of salt, if desired. Sauté, stirring frequently, until vegetables are barely tender, about 10 minutes.

Add crushed tomatoes, basil and oregano to taste, and a sprinkle of ground allspice. Squeeze in the garlic cloves. Simmer uncovered for 15 minutes. Meanwhile, grate the mozzarella and Parmesan.

Remove squash from pot or oven and allow to cool until you can handle it. If it is whole, cut it in half lengthwise, then remove seeds with a spoon and squeeze any excess water out of meat. Remove meat and break it up into strands with a fork or potato masher. Mix squash well with vegetables and put half in the bottom of a large baking dish. Top with half the cheeses, the rest of the squash, and then the rest of the cheeses.

Bake for 30 minutes or until cheese is bubbly and slightly browned. Let cool 15 to 20 minutes before serving.

Note:

Cheese can be omitted if needed.

Saffron Sea Bass with Potatoes and Bell Peppers (adapted from Ghillie Basan's Tagines and Couscous) (serves 8)

Good time to serve:

This is a lovely dish to serve when entertaining guests. However it can also be prepared on a weeknight, as it is simply baked in the oven.

Story behind this dish:

This dish became a favorite of mine when I started experimenting by cooking with tagines. These are beautiful one-pot cooking vessels that originate in Morocco. The secret to the tagine is that the food cooks gently in a small amount of liquid. The conical lid collects the steam and the water drips back onto the cooking food to seal in moisture and flavor. The dishes can be cooked in the oven or on the stove, and I love to use the tagine for cooking tender meats occasionally and of course vegetables and fish. I have collected two beautiful tagines and love throwing a tagine dinner party a few times a year.

Prep time: 20 minutes

Cook time: 60 minutes

Ingredients:

- *pinch of saffron threads*
- *⅔ cup warm water*
- *1 pound red potatoes*
- *4 large tomatoes, sliced*
- *6 cloves of garlic, peeled and smashed*
- *2 green bell peppers, cut into strips*
- *4 tbsp olive oil*
- *juice of 2 lemons*
- *2 pounds sea bass filet (can substitute any*

sustainable, wild-caught firm fish filet)

- 1 small preserved lemon cut into strips

- 2 tbsp sliced and pitted green olives

- handful of chopped cilantro

- handful of chopped parsley

- sea salt

- fresh ground black pepper

Directions:

Preheat oven to 350ºF.

First prepare the saffron. Dry-roast the threads in a small heavy bottom skillet for less than 1 minute. When you smell a faint aroma, remove them from the stove. Use a mortar and pestle or the back of a spoon to crush the threads into a powder. Add warm water until the saffron dissolves. Let this sit.

Line the base of an ovenproof deep dish (a tagine is preferable, but can also use a casserole-type dish or Dutch oven) with a layer of potatoes, topped with a layer of sliced tomatoes. Reserve a few slices of the tomatoes for the top of the fish. Scatter the garlic over the top, season with a little salt and pepper and arrange the bell peppers over the top. Reserve a few strips of bell pepper for the top of the fish. Pour half the prepared saffron water, half of the olive oil, and half of the lemon juice over the layers, cover and place in the preheated oven for about 25 minutes. The potatoes and bell peppers should be tender. Remove this from the oven.

Rub the sea bass (or selected fish) with a little salt and place it on top of the peppers. Mark the topside of the fish with 3 gashes and pour the rest of the saffron water, olive oil and lemon juice over the fish. Arrange the reserved tomato and bell pepper slices over the top of the fish and scatter the preserved lemon slices and olives over and around the fish. Cover the dish and return it to the oven for another 25 minutes, until the fish is just cooked.

Remove the lid and return the fish to the oven for the final 10 minutes. Sprinkle the chopped parsley and cilantro on top of the fish and serve it with warm crusty brown bread or plain couscous.

Notes:

If you are not familiar with preserved lemon, you can find it already prepared at markets such as Whole Foods, specialty middle-eastern food stores, Williams-Sonoma and even a farmer's market. It adds wonderful flavor to many dishes and can be kept in the fridge for months.

This dish features many healing and healthy ingredients: Fish is high in omega-3 fatty acids, necessary to help combat inflammation in our bodies and promote heart health. It's important to choose fish that is sustainable, wild or local caught, and as fresh as possible. The Monterey Bay Seafood Watch (**https://www.seafoodwatch.org/**) is a helpful guide. Additionally, the use of saffron in this dish is unique. Saffron is a highly flavorful spice that has potent anti-cancer antioxidants. Tomatoes are chock full of lycopene, a powerful antioxidant helpful in breast and prostate cancer prevention as well as prevention of Alzheimer's disease.

Crispy Brussel Sprouts with Garlic (serves 4-6)

Good time to serve:

I make this dish anytime for my family or friends. It is quick, and full of nutrients. My kids love it!

Story behind this dish:

As a kid, I loved Brussels sprouts. As an adult, I discovered that you could make Brussels sprouts crispy in the oven and they tasted so much better! I created this recipe to include lots of health-benefiting ingredients like ginger, garlic and sesame oil.

Prep time: 10 minutes

Cook time: 20 minutes

Ingredients:

- *1 pound Brussels sprouts, sliced in half*
- *¼ cup mirin*
- *2 tbsp shoyu or tamari (gluten-free soy sauce)*
- *1 inch peeled ginger root, grated*
- *3 cloves of minced garlic*
- *1 tsp maple syrup*
- *black pepper to taste*
- *2 tbsp toasted sesame oil*

Directions:

Preheat oven to 425°F.

Combine mirin, soy sauce, ginger, garlic and sugar (or maple syrup) in a small bowl. Toss over the Brussels sprouts and mix well. Spread on a large baking sheet, season with fresh black pepper, and roast in oven for 20 minutes until crispy.

Drizzle with toasted sesame oil.

Coconut Salmon Curry (serves 6)

Good time to serve:

This is a frequent dinner in our home. It is also a wonderfully hearty dish to serve to friends at a dinner party. During the summer if you want to lighten the dish, you can omit the coconut milk.

Story behind this dish:

I did not grow up eating a lot of fish in my house, as my father was not fond of it. My mother however grew up in a part of India where fish was a common part of the diet. She made one style of fish curry, and it typically included a firm white fish. I have adapted her recipe for salmon which is a typically found wild and is healthier. I also added a south Indian flair to this dish with the addition of coconut milk.

Cook time: 50 minutes

Ingredients:

- ¼ cup minced onion
- 3 large garlic cloves, minced
- 2 medium serrano chilies, minced
- 1½ tbsp minced fresh organic ginger
- ⅓ cup plus ¾ cup unsweetened coconut milk
- 3 tbsp coconut, avocado or thrive algae oil

- ½ tsp yellow mustard seeds
- 8 curry leaves, preferably fresh (see Note)
- 2 tsp ground fennel
- 1 tbsp ground coriander
- ¼ tsp ground cardamom
- ¼ tsp turmeric
- ¼ tsp cayenne pepper
- ⅔ cup water

- ½ cup chopped tomatoes
- 15 cherry tomatoes, halved
- 2 ¼ pounds skinless wild salmon fillet, cut into 1 ¼-inch chunks
- salt
- chopped cilantro for garnish

Directions:

In a mini food processor, combine the onion, garlic, serrano chilies and ginger with the ⅓ cup coconut milk and process to a paste. If ginger is organic, leave the skin on. This step can be prepared up to two days in advance and refrigerated.

In a cast iron or ceramic pot, heat the oil. Add the curry leaves and yellow mustard seeds and cook over moderately high heat until the seeds pop, about 1 minute. Add the coconut/ginger/onion paste and cook over moderate heat, stirring, until fragrant, about 4 minutes. Add the ground fennel, coriander, cardamom, turmeric, cayenne and cook, stirring, until fragrant, about 2 minutes. Add the remaining ¾ cup of coconut milk and the water, chopped tomatoes. Bring to a simmer, then bring heat to low and simmer over low heat for 10 minutes.

Add the cherry tomatoes to the sauce and simmer over moderate heat until just starting to soften, about 1 minute. Season the salmon with salt, add it to the skillet and simmer over moderate heat, gently stirring a few times, until just cooked through, about 3 minutes. Sprinkle with the chopped cilantro leaves and serve warm. This dish can be served with a cauliflower rice, quinoa or basmati rice.

Chocolate Avocado Mousse (serves 4-6)

Good time to serve:

This is a great dish for a weekday dessert or even a party. It is gluten free, dairy free, vegan and paleo which satisfies a lot of people! It is chock full of fiber, magnesium and healthy fats. Avocados also provide a great deal of potassium to your diet.

Story behind this dish:

I don't have much of a sweet tooth, but chocolate is one treat that I have a hard time resisting. This is a great way to satisfy my chocolate craving and get the health benefits. My kids also love this as an occasional dessert to enjoy.

Prep time: 30 minutes

Ingredients:

- *1 ounce organic 70%-100% cacao pure dark chocolate*
- *3 tbsp raw cacao powder*
- *3 tbsp coconut oil*
- *2 large ripe avocados, pitted (1½ cup) and smashed*
- *6 pitted medjool dates, soaked in warm water*
- *¼ cup coconut milk*
- *2 tbsp maple syrup*
- *1 tsp vanilla*

Directions:

Use a double boiler or put a small metal bowl or glass bowl on top of a smaller saucepan. The saucepan should be filled ¼ of the way with simmering water. Add the dark chocolate, raw cacao powder and coconut oil to the bowl so they melt together.

Add the avocado, dates, coconut milk, maple syrup and vanilla to a blender and blend until almost smooth. Add the melted chocolate mixture and blend until completely smooth. Place the mixture in separate bowls or one large bowl and chill in the refrigerator for four hours. This can also be eaten at room temperature. If storing the chocolate mousse for a longer period of time up to 2 days, cover it.

Egg Bhurji (Scrambled Eggs with Masala)

Good time to serve:

We eat a lot of eggs in our house, though we stick with no more than 7 per week per person. I have a difficult time eating scrambled eggs without spice. This dish is so satisfying, that it can be served for breakfast, in a breakfast taco, for lunch or for dinner. Typically, in India, it is served with a wheat roti or paratha (round, flat or layered unleavened bread).

Story behind this dish:

I grew up with this dish as staple in my house. Typically, it was served as breakfast, brunch or dinner. Sometimes it would be served with peas mixed in, and sometimes with spinach and tomatoes. The traditional style is with peas.

Prep time: 10 minutes

Cook time: 15 minutes

Ingredients:

- *6 eggs*
- *¼ cup fresh or frozen green peas*
- *1 medium onion, chopped*
- *1 medium tomato, chopped*
- *½ tsp coriander powder*
- *½ tsp cumin powder*
- *¼ tsp turmeric powder*
- *¼ tsp black pepper*
- *optional ½ tsp red chili powder and or 2 green chilies chopped*
- *2 tbsp butter*
- *¼ tbsp salt and to taste*
- *½ cup fresh cilantro chopped*

Directions:

Break the eggs into a bowl. Add the salt, coriander, cumin, turmeric, and black pepper (and chili pepper if using) to the bowl. Briskly whisk.

Heal the butter in a non-stick pan. Add the onions, and green chilies and sauté over medium heat until the onions are softened, about 10 minutes. Then add the tomatoes (and fresh green peas if using) and cook for another 5 minutes until tomatoes are softened. Then add the frozen green peas and cook for 3 minutes.

Add the beaten egg mixture to the pan and turn the heat to low. Gently stir the egg mixture, pulling it up from the bottom as it thickens. If you like your eggs soft and moist, remove them from the heat before they are fully dry as they will continue to cook after being removed from the pan.

Garnish the eggs with the chopped cilantro leaves.

Nani's Indian Spiced Turkey or Chicken Meatballs
(serves 4-6, total of 15-20 meatballs)

Good time to serve:

> This dish can be served for lunch, dinner or even as an appetizer at a cocktail party. It also makes a great finger food snack.

Story behind this dish:

> We call these meatballs kebabs in our house. Over many years, the recipe has changed and matured. It is a commonly found dish in the northern part of India, and you will find many variations of it. I learned this recipe from my mom also known as Nani (this means Grandma). I have adapted my current version of this recipe to suit the taste of my kids. It has a bit more moisture from yogurt, and tomato paste or ketchup and is typically made with less chilies. I also tend to add shredded carrots or zucchini to get a few more vegetables in their diet.

Prep time: 15 minutes

Cook time: 30

Ingredients:

- *1 pound of ground turkey or chicken (85% lean)*
- *1 tbsp chopped fresh garlic or paste*
- *1 tbsp ginger paste (fresh grated ginger also works)*
- *½ onion chopped finely*
- *1 egg*
- *1 tbsp of tomato paste*
- *option for 1 tbsp of organic ketchup (kids love this flavor)*
- *3-4 tbsp of yogurt (gauge the wetness of the meat as you don't want it too wet)*
- *½ tsp ground coriander*
- *½ tsp ground cumin*
- *¾ tsp kosher salt*

- ½ tsp fresh ground pepper
- 2 tbsp almond flour or meal or another gluten-free "breadcrumb" option
- 2 tbsp finely chopped fresh cilantro
- option for ½ cup shredded zucchini or carrots
- ½ tsp chili powder (use more for spicier meatballs)
- 2 tbsp of coconut, avocado, organic safflower, or thrive algae oil

Directions:

Preheat oven to 400 degrees Fahrenheit.

Combine all ingredients in a bowl together and mix and mash well. Shape these into balls or usually small oblong kebabs and set aside until they are all rolled.

Heat two tablespoons of oil on a skillet over medium heat until the oil is hot, but not smoking.

Pan fry the kebabs in batches to brown on each side, setting them aside on a paper-towel lined plate until they are all done. Approximately 5 to 7 minutes.

Then space them an inch or so apart on a lined baking sheet and bake in oven at 400 degrees for around 8-9 minutes.

Simple Broccoli

Good time to serve:

This is a frequent dinner side in our home. It is also a wonderfully light dish to serve as a side dish at a dinner party. During the summer if you want to lighten the dish, you can omit the coconut milk.

Story behind this dish:

Broccoli is a powerhouse vegetable and contains the largest concentrations of health-promoting sulfur compounds, sulforaphane and isothiocyanates, essential in liver detox. It also is rich in phytonutrients such as lutein and zeaxanthin which help with vision. Broccoli is also a potent provider of folic acid, vitamins A and C and fiber. Both florets and stem have high nutrient content, so I include both in this dish. If broccoli is overcooked, it begins to lose its nutrients, up to 50%. The ideal way to cook broccoli is to steam it. Additionally, studies show that the enzyme myrosinase which converts some of the plant nutrients into their active forms is released when broccoli is cut into smaller pieces. Allowing the broccoli to sit for 5-10 minutes allows the myrosinase to do its' job before the cooking heat destroys it. Vitamin C (found in lemon juice), mustard and turmeric increases myrosinase activity so sprinkling and of these on the broccoli helps concentrate the nutrients as well.

Ingredients:

- 1 pound of broccoli
- 2 medium cloves of garlic
- 2 tsp lemon juice
- 3 tbsp extra virgin olive oil
- optional spice mixture: garam masala, curry powder, tandoori powder (all of which contain turmeric) or Dijon mustard
- sea salt and pepper to taste

Directions:

Fill the bottom of a steamer or a pan with 2 inches of water. While the water is warming to a boil, cut the broccoli florets into quarters and let them sit. Cut the stems into ¼ inch pieces. Press or chop garlic and let it sit for 5 minutes.

Add the broccoli florets and stems to the steamer basket and sprinkle with the optional spice mixture. Steam for no more than 5 minutes. Transfer to a bowl. Toss the broccoli with the olive oil, lemon juice and pressed or chopped garlic or Dijon mustard and gently mix.

BONUS
CULINARY PHARMACY

Let Food Be Thy Medicine

Culinary medicine has emerged as an exciting blend of the art of food and cooking with evidence based medicine. The focus is on the use of foods in synergistic ways to improve patient outcomes and prevent disease. There are numerous reasons as to why nutritional science has evolved in this way.

The first is that there is widespread dissatisfaction with the lack of inclusion of a real understanding of nutrition in conventional medical practice. You might have found yourself in the position of asking your own doctor how you might eat better to control your symptoms or improve your health and have been provided little actionable information. The second reason is that there is a flourishing interest in popular cooking shows, cookbooks and food festivals as well as often conflicting popular dietary advice. There is also a revival of home gardening, local agriculture and farmer's markets that has revitalized the enthusiasm around additive-free local and organic food. Counter that with the growing number of fast food restaurants and convenient food items that lack nutritional value or have hidden ingredients that are adding to our society getting sicker, and fatter.

I strongly believe that you have to arm yourself with the knowledge to make decisions that benefit you and not rely on the food and beverage corporations or government recommendations to stay healthy, strong and thrive. I have studied culinary medicine at the Goldring Center for Culinary Medicine at Tulane University, taken years of evidence based nutritional education and I actively participate in organizations that support our local food system and increase access to quality food. I do all of this so that I can empower you to care for yourself by using healing foods, spices and herbs in beneficial ways and to have fun doing so.

Below, you will find a list of some of my favorite healing foods, spices and herbs and the health benefits listed. This list is not comprehensive as I could write a book on the number of foods that fit this category! Perhaps, that's an idea for my next book?

My desire is that you are encouraged to consider how you cook and enjoy food in a new way.

Perhaps understanding that many plants have a multitude of ways in which they nourish us will foster gratitude for the variety of vegetables, fruits, and herbs that are available to us as well as increase your palate. If you stop and think of it, plants communicate with every cell in our body via the nutrients they provide us. They rely on us for their survival as well to cultivate and spread them. Thus, we have a symbiotic relationship that has evolved over the course of human evolution. Enjoy and celebrate your food and most of all realize that you have powerful medicine available to you right in your own fridge or garden! Here's my quick-reference guide to the nutrients you need to pack into your diet pronto! It contains my best suggestions for foods you can use as medicine.

1. **Cruciferous vegetables**

   These include broccoli, cabbage, cauliflower, Brussels sprouts, kale, bok choy. They contain indoles (indole-3-carbinol) and flavones. Large studies show reduced breast cancer risk through I-3-c affecting estrogen metabolism, reduced lung, stomach and colorectal cancer risk. Indoles help maintain the levels of vitamins A, C, E in the body.

   How to obtain indoles from your cruciferae:

   - chopping and chewing your vegetable release glucosinolates which react with an enzyme to release indoles

   - don't boil these vegetables, because it affects the absorption of indoles

   - steaming is the ideal method to cook cruciferous vegetables

2. **Omega-3 fatty acids and Other Healthy Fats**

   Nuts and olive oil are great, because daily nut consumption can reduce mortality by one-fifth according to the New England Journal of Medicine. Nuts include walnuts, macadamia nuts, brazil nuts and almonds. Seeds such as flax and pumpkin seeds and seed oils are an important source of healthy fats. Other sources of healthy fats include avocado, olives and olive oil. You can also get omega-3 fatty acids from fatty fish like sockeye salmon or wild fish such as sardines, trout, mackerel and halibut. Omega-3 fatty acids help nerve cells communicate well with each other. This supports good mental health.

Healthy fats also help reduce cortisol (stress hormone) levels. The greatest effect that omega-3 fatty acids have on your body is its' powerful anti-inflammatory effect.

3. Grapes/Red Wine

These colorful foods contain resveratrol, a polyphenolic phytonutrient, and anthocyanins. They have positive effects on cognitive function, heart conditions, cancer, and decrease inflammation. If you currently do not drink alcohol, there is no reason to start. However, if you do, then choose red wine for its powerful health benefits. Stick to the guidelines of no more than one glass of wine per day for women, and no more than two glasses of wine per day for men.

4. Colorful Berries

Darkly colored fruits like blueberries, raspberries, goji berries, elderberries, and blackberries contain antioxidants. Antioxidants help reduce free radicals (toxic chemicals produced when under stress), which cause damage to the body and increase the aging process. These berries also protect against heart disease, stroke, and vision loss from macular degeneration and cataracts.

5. Flax/Sesame Seeds

Lignans are found in the woody portion of plants. Flaxseed and sesame seeds (335 mg and 373 mg per 100g respectively) have lignan content a hundred times higher than other dietary sources and are a great dietary resource for this phytonutrient. Lignans help block the effects of estrogen and therefore may be beneficial in reducing the risk or estrogen associated cancers such as breast, uterine and ovarian cancers. In fact, research has also shown that post-menopausal women who regularly intake lignans through their diet have a 15% reduced risk of breast cancer.

6. Tomato and Red Fruits and Vegetables

These contain lycopene which is one of the most potent antioxidants and has been suggested to prevent the growth of cancer and heart disease by protecting critical biomolecules including lipids, low-density lipoproteins (LDL), proteins and DNA.

7. Green Tea

Contains flavonoids including Epigallocatechin gallate (EGCG). Green tea has been found to decrease mortality from all causes, including cardiovascular disease, diabetes, some cancers.

8. Dark Chocolate

Great news! Dark chocolate has protective effects on heart disease, and breast cancer as well as other health benefits. Be sure your chocolate is at least 70% cacao to reap the benefits. There are various chocolates on the market that are also paleo-friendly and thus have used stevia as a natural sweetener instead of processed sugar. Also, I suggest making sure your chocolate is organic to avoid pesticides, and other harmful chemicals found in non-organic chocolate.

9. Fermented Foods/Beneficial Bacteria

Beneficial bacteria help with the absorption of nutrients from food, immunity, detoxification, and with the breakdown of complex carbohydrates.

They also create a mucous barrier between the interior of the gut and the lining of the intestines. The bacteria in our gut influence everything from mood and behavior to how we control our weight to our cravings for certain foods. Having fermented foods in your diet such as yogurt, kefir, sauerkraut, and pickled vegetables help keep the variety of gut bugs healthy. It's also important to feed these guys with prebiotic foods such as onions, garlic, artichoke and fiber from a variety of vegetables and fruits.

10. Garlic

Garlic acts as both an antibacterial as well as an anti-fungal. It also has many cardiovascular benefits including decreasing risk of heart disease, stroke and lowering cholesterol. There are over 3000 studies on garlic, many of them also showing a decreased risk of colon cancer with daily consumption. Garlic should be crushed, pressed or chopped to expose the potent compound allicin which is responsible for many of its health benefits. It should sit for about 10 minutes exposed to the air and then eaten raw or added at the end of cooking to a dish with fat. One clove a day is all that's needed to reap the benefits of this superfood.

BONUS:
SPICE PHARMACY

Your Medicinal Pantry

1. Turmeric

Curcumin (beneficial chemical found in turmeric) is a powerful antioxidant, anti-inflammatory agent and inducer of cell cycle arrest (which means it helps stop cancer growth). It's a root spice that is boiled, dried and made into powder. Powdered turmeric contains 3% curcumin by weight.

It decreases arthritic pain, Alzheimer's disease and inflammatory bowel disease. Unfortunately, it's not very bioavailable, which means that the body doesn't absorb it well, unless it's taken with black pepper (piperine) and fat.

Use in recipes featuring: curries, lentils, soups, vegetables especially cauliflower and tomatoes.

2. Cumin

This spice helps protect bones, decreasing osteoporosis risk. It also helps regulate blood sugar, and decreases risk of diabetes related cataract progression.

It decreases formation of AGE (advanced glycation end products) by 40-90%. AGEs contribute to the aging process and are created when foods are cooked over high heat. The volatile oil of cumin contains vitamins C and A. It also acts in cancer prevention and as an anti-microbial (especially against food poisoning).

Use in recipes featuring: black beans, chili, curries, Mexican food, tomatoes.

3. Coriander

This spice is made up of 85% volatile oils, two of which (linalool and geranyl acetate) are antioxidants. It improves IBS symptoms, constipation, and protects against ulcers. Typical medicinal use of coriander is for digestive complaints, loss of appetite, bloating, flatulence and cramps. Coriander oil can sooth eczema, psoriasis, rosacea. It also helps in diabetes, decreases LDL, and increases HDL.

Use in recipes featuring: beans, fish, lentils, vegetables, any meats.

4. Caraway

Contains carvone which relaxes digestive spasms. Also contains limonene, which inhibits breast, liver, lung and stomach cancer. Inhibits the growth of E. Coli bacteria which can cause infectious diarrhea.

Use in recipes featuring: apples, cheese, potatoes, onion tarts.

5. Ginger

Helps with indigestion through increasing pancreatic digestive enzymes. It is an effective antinausea agent, and helps with osteoarthritic pain. In cancer therapy, it activates tumor suppressor genes and down-regulates a gene involved in metastasis thereby helping to prevent the spread of cancer.

Use in recipes featuring: chicken, winter squashes, duck, shellfish and sweet potatoes, add to smoothies.

6. Cinnamon

Helps with blood sugar control and diabetes. It is also effective in helping symptoms of polycystic ovarian syndrome by helping with managing insulin and blood sugar spikes. This spice is also an anti-microbial and anti-fungal.

Be sure to use Cinnamomum verum (true cinnamon) also called Ceylon cinnamon for its' increased health benefits. Ceylon cinnamon contains antioxidant compounds called proanthocyanadins which strengthen blood vessels and protect the body from damage by UV radiation. This type of cinnamon can be found in specialty spice shops or Indian marketplaces. Its appearance has rolled thinner multilayers compared to the thicker bark of cassia cinnamon. All types of cinnamon contain cinnamaldehyde which is the active ingredient.

Use in recipes featuring: curries, winter squash, apples, pastries, bananas, chicken, Moroccan tagine, cauliflower.

7. Black Cumin Seed (Nigella Satva)

This spice has a unique antioxidant called thymoquinone. It has been shown to boost immunity, lower blood pressure, decrease cholesterol and decrease heart disease. It has been found to be a potent anti-cancer agent, halting the growth and spread of tumors. Additionally, black cumin seed extract can decrease symptoms of asthma and allergies.

Use in recipes featuring: chutneys, lamb, chocolate, rice, potatoes and mangos.

8. Cloves

Eugenol is the aromatic and powerful oil in clove. It is responsible for the numbing effect that clove oil has on gums and mouth tissue and can be rubbed around a painful tooth. It is an anti-inflammatory, an analgesic and an antibacterial. It has germ-fighting properties that have been noted in combatting H.Pylori and herpes simplex. It also has the ability to act as an anti-clotting agent to stop blood clots forming in your arteries.

Use in recipes featuring: pumpkin, apples, chocolate, cabbage, Indian cuisine, and cabbage.

9. Rosemary

This is a spice to get familiar with. High heat used for cooking meats, including grilling, broiling, frying and smoking cause an accumulation of toxic compounds in the meat. Adding rosemary extract to your grilled meats significantly reduces the levels of these harmful compounds. Rosemary has also been shown to be protective to the skin against UV damage, and supports the liver against liver damage from toxic chemicals. This spice also acts as an anti-inflammatory and helps with decreasing arthritic pain.

Use in recipes featuring: chicken, game, grilled vegetables, lamb, tomato sauces, pork.

10. Saffron

This is the world's most expensive spice. It is also a powerful antidepressant and helps maintain levels of brain chemicals involved in stabilizing and boosting mood. Saffron has many health benefits ranging from slowing mental decline in Alzheimer's disease to helping slow the progressing of macular degeneration.

Use in recipes featuring: chicken, tagine, couscous, rice, soups, lamb, curries and puddings.

ABOUT
SHELLY SETHI

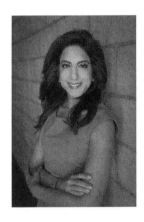

Dr. Sethi brings her trailblazing program to patients all over the world. She believes that health is a journey and manifests through a balance of nutrition, environment, community, spirituality, mindset and physical movement. She offers individualized consultations, workshops, online webinars and seminars to anyone looking to transform their lives and regain their energy and vitality. Her mission is to offer practical, sustainable lifestyle interventions that focus on the root-cause of illness rather than providing a band-aid. She currently lives in Austin, Texas with her husband, also a practicing integrative medicine physician, and her two young boys.

Citations

Melatonin:

Kandil TS, Mousa AA, El-Gendy AA, Abbas AM. The potential therapeutic effect of melatonin in gastro-esophageal reflux disease. BMC Gastroenterology. 2010;10:7.

Torres JDFDO, Pereira RDS. Which is the best choice for gastroesophageal disorders: Melatonin or proton pump inhibitors? World J Gastrointest Pharmacol Ther 2010; 1(5): 102-106.

Sleep:

Zhu L, Zee PC. Circa`dian Rhythm Sleep Disorders. Neurologic clinics. 2012;30(4):1167-1191.

Sources cited:

http://time.com/3183183/best-time-to-sleep/

Obesity data:

Sources cited:

World Health Organization: http://www.who.int/news-room/fact-sheets/detail/obesity-and-overweight

Exercise:

Charatan F. Exercise and diet reduce risk of diabetes, US study shows. BMJ: British Medical Journal. 2001;323(7309):359.

Lindholm ME1, Marabita F, Gomez-Cabrero D, Rundqvist H, Ekström TJ, Tegnér J, Sundberg CJ.Epigenetics. 2014 Dec;9(12):1557-69.

Sharma A, Madaan V, Petty FD. Exercise for Mental Health. Primary Care Companion to The Journal of Clinical Psychiatry. 2006;8(2):106.

Otto MW, Church TS, Craft LL, Greer TL, Smits JAJ, Trivedi MH. Exercise for Mood and Anxiety Disorders. Primary Care Companion to The Journal of Clinical Psychiatry. 2007;9(4):287-294.

Social relationships and health:

JS House, KR Landis, D Umberson. Science 29 Jul 1988: Vol. 241, Issue 4865, pp. 540-545.

Social isolation:

Valtorta NK, Kanaan M, Gilbody S, *et al.* Loneliness and social isolation as risk factors for coronary heart disease and stroke: systematic review and meta-analysis of longitudinal observational studies. *Heart* 2016;102:1009-1016.

Loneliness and cognitive decline:

Wilson RS, Bennett DA. How Does Psychosocial Behavior Contribute to Cognitive Health in Old Age? Brain Sci. 23 May 2017, 7(6).

Boss L, Kang DH, Branson S. Loneliness and cognitive function in the older adult: a systematic review. International Psychogeriatrics. 02 Jan 2015, 27(4):541-553.

Barnes DE, Alexopoulos GS, Lopez OL, Williamson JD, Yaffe K. Depressive symptoms, vascular disease, and mild cognitive impairment: findings from the Cardiovascular Health Study. Arch. Gen. Psychiatry. 01 Mar 2006, 63(3):273-279.

Association of religious service attendance with mortality among women:

Shanshan Li, ScD, Meir J. Stampfer, MD, DrPH; David R. Williams, PhD;Tyler J. VanderWeele, PhD. *JAMA Intern Med.* 2016;176(6):777-785.

Mindfulness:

Singleton O, Hölzel BK, Vangel M, Brach N, Carmody J, Lazar SW. Change in Brainstem Gray Matter Concentration Following a Mindfulness-Based Intervention is Correlated with Improvement in Psychological Well-Being. *Frontiers in Human Neuroscience.* 2014;8:33.

Michael D. Mrazek, Michael S. Franklin, Dawa Tarchin Phillips, Benjamin Baird, and Jonathan W. Schooler. *Psychological Science.* Vol 24, Issue 5, pp. 776 - 781. March 28, 2013.

Other Sources Cited:

Chiasson, Ann Marie. *Energy Healing: The Essentials of Self-Care.* Boulder: Sounds True Inc., 2013. Print.

Buettner, D. (2012). *The blue zones: 9 lessons for living longer from the people who've lived the longest (2nd ed.)*. Washington, D.C.: National Geographic.

Aggarwal, B. B., & Yost, D. (2011). *Healing spices: How to use 50 everyday and exotic spices to boost health and beat disease*. New York: Sterling Pub. Co.

Weil, A., Fox, Sam. *True Food: Seasonal, Sustainable, Simple, Pure*. Little, Brown and Company; Reprint edition (April 1, 2014)

https://www.drweil.com/diet-nutrition/anti-inflammatory-diet-pyramid/dr-weils-anti-inflammatory-diet/

Made in the USA
San Bernardino, CA
08 November 2018